EUROPE'S LABORATORY

A volume in the

NIU Series in Slavic, East European, and Eurasian Studies

Edited by Christine D. Worobec

For a list of books in the series, visit our website at cornellpress.cornell.edu.

EUROPE'S LABORATORY

CLIMATE AND HEALTH IN EIGHTEENTH-CENTURY RUSSIA

MATTHEW P. ROMANIELLO

NORTHERN ILLINOIS UNIVERSITY PRESS
AN IMPRINT OF CORNELL UNIVERSITY PRESS

First published 2025 by Cornell University Press

Library of Congress Cataloging-in-Publication Data

Names: Romaniello, Matthew P., author.
Title: Europe's laboratory : climate and health in eighteenth-century Russia / Matthew P. Romaniello.
Description: Ithaca, New York : Northern Illinois University Press, an imprint of Cornell University Press, 2025. | Series: NIU series in Slavic, East European, and Eurasian studies | Includes bibliographical references and index.
Identifiers: LCCN 2025003332 (print) | LCCN 2025003333 (ebook) | ISBN 9781501783920 (hardcover) | ISBN 9781501783937 (epub) | ISBN 9781501783944 (pdf)
Subjects: LCSH: Medical climatology—Russia—History—18th century. | Medical geography—Russia—History—18th century. | Medicine—Research—History—18th century. | Public health—Russia—History—18th century. | Public health—Research—History—18th century.
Classification: LCC RA877 .R55 2025 (print) | LCC RA877 (ebook) | DDC 613/.110947—dc23 /eng/20250529
LC record available at https://lccn.loc.gov/2025003332
LC ebook record available at https://lccn.loc.gov/2025003333

Contents

Abbreviations

BA	Bedfordshire Archives, Bedford, Great Britain
BRB	Beinecke Rare Book and Manuscript Library, Yale University, New Haven, CT
BL	The British Library, Manuscripts, London
LCR	Library Carolina Rediviva, University of Uppsala, Sweden
NLS	National Library of Scotland, Special Collections, Edinburgh
NRS	National Records of Scotland, Edinburgh
PSZ	*Polnoe sobranie zakonov Rossiiskoi Imperii*
RSA	Royal Society for the Arts Archive, London
TNA	The National Archives, Kew, Richmond, Surrey, Great Britain
WL	Wellcome Library, Rare Materials, London

Note on Transliteration, Spelling, and Dates

The transliteration of Russian words and names follows the Library of Congress system except for the familiar spelling of the tsars, including Peter I, Catherine II, and Paul I, and familiar cities, including St. Petersburg and Moscow. The spelling of original sources has been retained for the English sources. Dates on all documents are given as listed in the original sources, although I have adjusted some to reflect January 1 as the start of a new year. In 1752, Britain switched to the Gregorian calendar. Documents following that date written by British diplomats in Russia tend to have two dates, reflecting the Russian and British calendars. In those cases, both dates are indicated in the notes.

Introduction

Tsar Alexander I's personal physician, Alexander Crichton, arrived in Russia from Britain in 1803 and would go on to serve the tsar for two decades. In the wake of Napoleon's invasion, Crichton published an account of an experimental treatment for consumption he had developed during his time in the capital. Crichton's study offered an answer as to how Russia's subjects remained so healthy in a land known for its extremely cold weather, which recently devastated the Grande Armée. Crichton acknowledged: "Consumption is infinitely more frequent in Great Britain and Ireland, in comparison of their population, than in the northern parts of Russia, yet the climate of Russia is in general infinitely colder and ruder than ours." Not only was the disease less common than expected but also Russian peasants recovered from consumption at a better rate than the British did. Crichton explained: "Whether this arises from the constant warmth in which the Russian lives, the frequent use of his vapour bath, or from the poverty of his diet, I do not pretend to say, but the fact is so; and to this difference of constitution, and other adventitious circumstances to be mentioned hereafter, the greater success in curing this class of patients may, perhaps, be owing."[1] Crichton also acknowledged that Russia's climate was dangerous, but he was confident that Russia's peasants had adapted successfully to its environment.

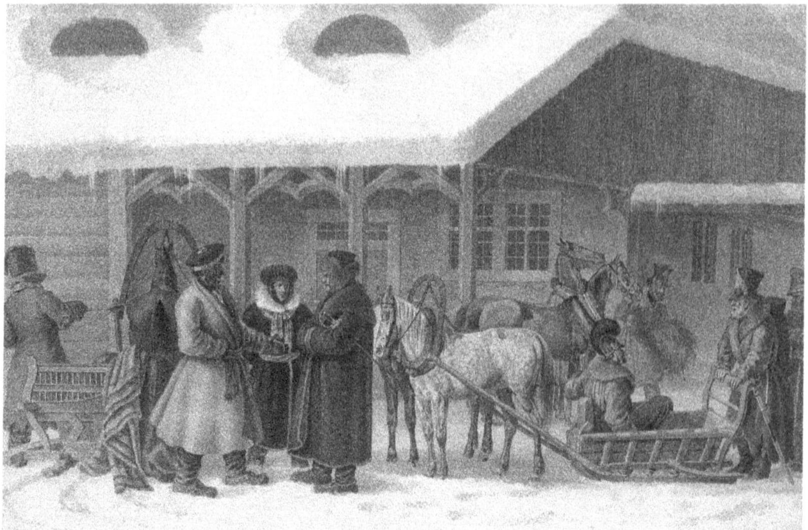

FIGURE I.1. Christian Wilhelm von Faber du Faur, "Between Braunsberg and Elbing. Officers and soldiers of Napoleon's Grand Armée with a sleigh outside an inn," in *Blaetter aus meinem Portfeuille, im Laufe des Feldzugs 1812 in Russland* (Stuttgart: C. F. Autenrieth, 1831–1834). From the British Library Archive.

Crichton expected his audience to understand that Britain had a temperate climate but that leaving its shores for any distant land meant exposure to intemperate conditions, risking one's health. Crichton accepted this idea, documenting Russia's dangerous climate while noting the Russians' ability to thrive in this extreme environment. An intemperate climate, in fact, offered an opportunity for those adapted to its distinct aspects, whereas those who were unsuited to it, as the French army had been, suffered and died from the same conditions (figure I.1).

Climate and health were linked concepts before Crichton wrote at the dawn of the nineteenth century, as it was an intrinsic part of the prevailing medical system, humoral theory. Climate and health had been associated as early as Hippocrates's well-known *On Airs, Waters, and Places* and was adopted and expanded on by Galen's time in classical Rome. Crichton, like most physicians working in the long eighteenth century, relied on a more recent advocate of the theory, the famous English physician Thomas Sydenham. Sydenham published extensively on his investigation of the causes of diseases in the late seventeenth century; his ideas would inspire a system of disease classification that would be known as nosology. Sydenham argued that understanding climatological conditions was necessary to understand disease outbreaks. In fact, these conditions may have been the most important aspect: "We must confess, that the above-mention'd Qualities of the Air do more or less dispose our Bodies to generate this or that Epidemick Disease." He claimed certain endemic diseases recurred in particular seasons, because of seasonal climate changes. For the British, he explained, measles and malaria appeared in January or February, "yet they also withdraw at the approach of the Summer Solstice. But others that begin in the Spring increase daily, and do not come to their State till the Autumnal Aequinox, which being past, they begin to retreat, and at length are extinguish'd by the cold of Winter. Of this kind is the Plague and Small-Pox, in those Years they are Epidemical."[2] Sydenham's association of season and disease may seem unscientific to a modern audience, but his nosological categorization of diseases underlay the medical curriculum for more than a century following its publication. Every physician working in the Russian Empire in the eighteenth century, including Crichton at the dawn of the nineteenth, was familiar with the principle that climate and health were linked and accepted that certain climates produced disease in specific seasons.

Crichton's publication recorded his clinical trials to treat consumption. Every spring, he observed, a consumption outbreak arrived in St. Petersburg. Consumption, like all pulmonary conditions, was known to be a "cold disease," in other words, a disease produced by a cold climate.[3] Plague outbreaks were not unknown in Russia, occurring three times in the eighteenth century alone, but medical authorities in the empire argued for a minimal response, quite confident that the arrival of winter would defeat an improbable hot disease inside the empire.[4] More attention was always paid to the endemic disease burden, particularly scurvy, syphilis, and smallpox. The Russian Empire as a whole, with its great northern expanse, regularly produced outbreaks of scurvy, arguably the best-known cold disease of the eighteenth century.[5] Syphilis was declared more than once to be unsolvable because suffering from a hot disease (as it was centered on a man's genitals, the source of a body's heat) in a cold climate meant the environment could not offer any effective treatment. When Russia began its smallpox inoculation trials after 1768, however, it offered a glimmer of hope for untreatable diseases. As inoculation expanded, the empire took its first important steps to improve the health of its subjects. If smallpox could be managed, could new solutions for scurvy and syphilis be far behind?

An increasing numbers of studies have examined Europe's encounters and adaptations to hot climates in the early modern era, including Karen Ordahl Kupperman's work on the Atlantic world and Mark Harrison's study of India.[6] Europeans emigrated from temperate conditions at home to intemperate climates in the Caribbean, sub-Saharan Africa, and South Asia. English settlers in the Caribbean, for example, considered surviving malaria a necessary "seasoning" process to become adapted to unhealthy conditions.[7] The Atlantic slave trade was motivated in part by the European certainty that African bodies were better suited toward labor in tropical climates.[8] Russia offered European empires an intriguing counterstudy: what happened in an extremely cold climate? Physicians at work in Europe wrote to their colleagues in Russia with questions on the health challenges of the cold empire. Physicians working in Russia published their case notes and observations in multiple languages across Europe as proof of their expertise on the topic. When Crichton wrote about consumption in 1823, part of the task was to prove that Russia had mastered another endemic challenge.

Writing about climate and health in the Russian Empire over the long eighteenth century, therefore, is as much about European global colonial strategies as it is about Russia specifically. The empire offered physicians a specialized laboratory that could inform ongoing discussions about health and disease. For the British at work in the Russian Empire, the most prominent of whom were the tsar's personal physicians like Crichton, information from Russia only gained greater currency after the British acquisition of Canada from France following the Seven Years' War. In other words, working within the Russian Empire assisted not only the Russian government by improving health outcomes for its subjects but also other colonial projects. Imperial science did not stop at geographic borders.

Sharing Knowledge, Improving Empire

The early modern era was defined, in part, by two linked processes: European expansion with its goal of empire-building; and the climatological crisis of the Little Ice Age and its influence on the lived experiences of people around the globe, including recurring famines and pandemics. The Little Ice Age extended from the fourteenth to the early nineteenth century, but the 1630s and 1640s were particularly traumatic in the northern hemisphere. The nadir of solar radiation reaching the Earth, combined with multiple massive volcanic eruptions in Southeast Asia, led to one of the coldest decades in centuries. Famines were rampant throughout Europe, causing multiple disease outbreaks, including typhus and the plague. The years 1648 and 1649 were rife with global political revolts, several of which began as food riots that expanded into other complaints against inadequate governments.[9] Russia was not immune to these effects, with riots against the tsar beginning in Moscow in 1648 and spreading as far away as Siberia in 1649.[10] Russia's political upheaval was followed by a plague outbreak in the mid-1650s, which also was linked to poor health from limited food supplies.[11]

What historians might conclude was a logical connection between climatological disasters and political and social consequences was not clear to contemporaries living in this era. Observing a lengthy winter or cool summer was not immediately connected to a disease outbreak at the time, but the unpredictable weather of that era provides an explanation of why discussions of the climate were so common among European writers. Although interest in the Little Ice Age and its consequences on historical events has been increasing in the modern era, much of what has been published has approached the issue as a particular colonial challenge. The surprise of leaving Britain and arriving in a different climate, particularly a warmer climate, frequently featured in British travel narratives to the colonies. In the eighteenth century, Britain's massive acquisition of Canada from France at the end of the Seven Years' War sparked a new curiosity about the challenges of leaving temperate Britain for a notably cold region. The health challenges for Canadian settlers were necessarily different than those for Jamaican or South African colonizers.[12]

British physicians had a long experience of living in a cold space to draw on—the Russian Empire. Following the English arrival in Russia in the sixteenth century, the tsars frequently hired English and Scottish physicians for the court.[13] Well positioned at the center of the Russian Empire, physicians and naturalists in Britain did not hesitate to ask their colleagues working in Moscow, and later St. Petersburg, for advice on the experience of cold. Robert Boyle relied on Tsar Aleksei Mikhailovich's doctor, Samuel Collins, to conduct experiments on the consequences of cold temperatures on air pressure in the 1650s.[14] When Dr. James Lind was completing his famous *Treatise on Scurvy* in 1753, he similarly relied on another British physician in Russia, John Cook, for his expert knowledge from having treated multiple disease outbreaks while working as a military physician in the Baltic Region.[15]

Once Britain acquired Canada in 1763, the interest in cold climates was no longer a scientific curiosity but rather an imperial necessity.

Russia and Canada may have been understood by the British as cold spaces, but without question, the focus of most European empires was squarely placed on even warmer and tropical environments. Britain, France, Spain, Portugal, and the Netherlands may have each taken part in Europe's expansion across the Atlantic and into the Indian Ocean, but their common interest was commercial products. The perception was that tropical agricultural products and Asian finished goods were more valuable than the potential exports from cold environments. The reality is the British Russia Company was the second-most-profitable British trading company in the eighteenth century, after the East India Company, but far ahead of all the others.[16] Historians have generally followed the expressed interest of their sources in the seventeenth and eighteenth centuries into tropical climates rather than into the colder ones. This has been important work, but it is simply impossible to understand the consequences of Europe's colonial ambitions without considering a more inclusive approach that accommodates all of Europe's entanglements.

This goal of this book, therefore, is to situate Russia and its imperial subjects as part of the ongoing discussions of Europe's empires. The Russian Empire was valued in scientific and medical circles as a distinct environment that offered expansive opportunities for observation and bioprospecting, both of which contributed to knowledge of the natural world.[17] The numerous publications by Russia's physicians that appeared in Britain, France, and Germany, among other countries, demonstrates the value of this project across Europe. Russia's physicians and naturalists did not operate outside of the main events of European history, but rather were active and integrated participants.

The physicians and naturalists working in Russia contributed to several key debates in early-modern Europe that influenced colonial enterprises, not only climate and geography but also health and demographic challenges, both for settlers and the Indigenous communities. One of the recurring issues in understanding the material generated by imperial observers is the way this knowledge was mediated through European, and frequently West European, lenses. Numerous authors have considered critically the ways this knowledge was produced and conceptualized to fit within existing frames of reference and hierarchies.[18] Postcolonial approaches to Western knowledge offer some opportunities to revisit and rethink the language chosen and how certain ideas were embedded, including a turn toward racialization as the eighteenth century progressed.[19] Important consideration has also been given to how Western observers could sexualize the objects of their encounter.[20] None of these texts can be taken at face value.

Even with reasonable concerns about the preconceptions, misinformation, and outright bias against non-Western subjects, physicians and naturalists working in this era made significant contributions toward the production of new scientific and medical information.[21] In an Atlantic context, it is unsurprising how the construction of race and its explicit connection to the exploitation of unfree labor has received the most attention.[22] Considering the work of this community of physicians in Russia in the same era provides an opportunity to reevaluate this Atlantic work by understanding its impact in a different racial and ethnic context, particularly as it was generated by the multiple peoples living across the vast expanse of Siberia.

In the eighteenth century, the Russian Empire was unquestionably one of the world's largest by area, albeit with a smaller population than most of the other European empires and even further behind the great empires of Asia. European perception of a population gap posed a significant challenge for Russian authorities, who encountered regular criticism of Russia's empty or barren spaces. Settler colonialism could offer an opportunity to work this land and exploit the empire's numerous resources, but the Russian government did not suddenly embrace a freedom of movement for its subjects.[23] If anything, the state became increasingly restrictive following the formalization of enserfment in 1649 until the loosening of these legal regulations in the middle of the nineteenth century. When foreign critics of the empire remarked on its emptiness, this was a result not only of a health crisis, a difficult climate, and a stretched food supply but also of the legal and social reality of the Russian state. To a degree, this can make it difficult to separate commentary on Russian politics, economic structures, and imperial government from debates about health and climate; these issues were connected. Ample historiographical discussions exist, however, on the tsars, society, and politics, and even important interventions for the problematic observations of contemporary Europeans on those issues.[24] This book, therefore, does not need to reassess these thoroughly studied topics but rather will focus on the two issues yet to be fairly examined: climate and health. It builds on a small but important historiography, including studies by Ryan Tucker Jones and Hans

Vermeulen, who have published the work of the Academy of Sciences and their foreign experts in the period.[25]

The Academy of Sciences, however, is not the central institution of this study but rather one of the employers of this book's actual subjects—the physicians who were working in Russia during the eighteenth century and their public health interventions.[26] Although earlier studies examined the history of medicine in Russia in the eighteenth century, those scholars did not approach the topic as a colonial issue.[27] The exception is Clare Griffin's work, but her focus is on pharmaceutical products and trade rather than on settler colonialism or disease outbreaks.[28] Extensive work on the effects of the cold climate on Russia's populations also remains lacking.[29]

There is an established history for the idea of public health in the eighteenth century as part of the Enlightenment project. It would not be until 1776 when the English philosopher Jeremy Bentham argued that achieving the "greatest happiness for the greatest number that is the measure of right and wrong," but this principal underlay many of the ideas circulating throughout the Enlightenment.[30] The application of reason to social problems, in theory, produced greater happiness for society. The application of new ideas in science and medicine to produce better health outcomes follows the same principle. Improving the health of the empire, and increasing the size of its population, were common goals across Europe. Considering how these goals were accomplished in a cold empire during the Little Ice Age, however, is a unique story.

The Cold Empire

This book is a study of climate, health, and empire, but it examines how these issues were framed by the public discussions in the eighteenth century. Therefore, I begin with an analysis of a particular system of rhetoric, promoted through a series of published narratives in the long eighteenth century. It is an analysis of the development of medical and scientific knowledge in consideration of how these ideas were mediated by an established system of rhetoric relied on by physicians and naturalists. It is not a book about class, gender, or nationality, although literacy was a prerequisite for participation in the system of rhetoric that tends to reify the importance of wealth and status. This system of rhetoric was based on humoral principles, which continued to define peoples and spaces long after scientists became more skeptical about the scientific validity of those ideals. The public, and published, discussion was led by physicians and naturalists, some working for the Russian government at the Academy of Sciences and the College of Medicine, but some outside the empire offering more pointed critiques. A private, and unpublished, discussion paralleled the other, led by diplomats and merchants working inside the Russian Empire, who attempted to describe and understand its populations.

The exchange of knowledge in the public and private spheres was not separate. The physician Johann Amman, for example, was one of the first botanists of the Russian Academy of Sciences. He published his research on Russia's and Siberia's plants, highlighting their distinct ability to survive cold temperatures. He relied on British merchants to exchange his Russian materials with the Royal Society in London. Those merchants worked both for themselves and for the British government, slipping in and out of the role of British consul to the Russian court. Johann Georg Gmelin, a physician and botanist working for the Russian Academy as part of the Second Kamchatka Expedition (1733–1743), published a narrative of the expedition and his multivolume *Flora Sibirica*, while privately debating with Dr. Carl Linnaeus about his new taxonomic system. Amman and Gmelin, therefore, both participated in a public discussion about science and health and privately corresponded with key figures across Europe.

Part 1 of the book considers the way the production of knowledge was limited by the choice of men who worked for the empire and the way in which they were educated; these limits tended to produce familiar types of information for an established audience. Chapter 1 unpacks the rhetoric that the medical and scientific community used to describe the peoples, lands, and environments of Russia. Although eighteenth-century science had evolved from traditional humoral ideas, physicians, and physicians working as naturalists, relied on the language of humoralism to denote the importance of climate, diet, activity and rest, and sex and reproduction (the so-called nonnaturals). The resulting observations expected an audience who understood the significance of this specific idiom. This first chapter documents the evolution of the naturalists' rhetoric that inscribed a certain type of medical knowledge on the body of the tsar's subjects. Russia was a cold place, as much as the empire's specialists may have resisted the label. European scientists accordingly turned toward Russia as a laboratory for cold experiments.

Chapter 2 discusses the evolution of the medical curriculum and practice from traditional humoral theory to incorporate innovations in anatomy, chemistry, and botany, including the implementation of Dr. Herman Boerhaave's medical curriculum at Leiden. Physicians and naturalists working in Russia were trained in Boerhaave's system, creating a body of knowledge that became the foundation of health interventions in the empire. By connecting a collective biography of the physicians working for the Russian state with the medical curriculum that produced their knowledge, this chapter highlights overlapping personal and educational networks that created a select group of professionals whose work defined the operation of empire. This group guided the ongoing debates about climate and health for the next century.

Part 2 moves beyond the established information networks to consider the ways in which the knowledge these men produced was implemented, not only in Russia but also across Europe and its empires. Empress Catherine I, Peter the Great's widow, opened the Russian Academy of Sciences in 1725. It provided the leadership for the Second Kamchatka Expedition, the scientific expedition in which Vitus Bering mapped the Strait that would later be named in his honor. Chapter 3 uses the establishment of the academy and the rich ethnographic texts produced by the expedition to explore Russia's contribution toward Carl Linnaeus's new taxonomic system. The Second Kamchatka Expedition became defined by its struggles to manage scurvy, which resulted in Bering's death among numerous others. By searching for local remedies across the empire and gathering extensive data on the progress of the disease, Russia's ability to manage its recurring scurvy outbreaks was established across Europe. In Britain, as James Lind prepared his famous *Treatise of Scurvy*, he corresponded with a colleague in Russia to uncover the latest information on the disease. By the middle of the eighteenth century, in other words, Russia's medical establishment was contributing actively to ongoing taxonomic and medical research in Sweden and Britain.

If its contributions to scurvy reflected a breakthrough, setbacks quickly followed. Foreign critics, primarily from France, published a series of attacks in the middle of the century, outlining the ongoing danger of Russia's climate on the health of its population. In 1761, Jean-Baptiste Chappe d'Auteroche, one of the few Frenchmen ever to conduct scientific work in early-modern Russia, published a scathing assessment of Russia's mismanagement of its peoples and resources. In 1762, Catherine the Great's coup not only overthrew her husband but also marked the beginning of her active involvement of repudiating the claims of Chappe d'Auteroche. In quick succession, Catherine's government laid out a new medical curriculum in her famous *Instruction*, required the Academy of Sciences to launch an extensive translation program to make major scientific and medical works available in Russian to the literate public, and even used her own body as a site for an experimental procedure—smallpox variolation. Chapter 4 analyzes the method by which Catherine's government implemented a series of health interventions to increase the size of Russia's population.

If Catherine's smallpox campaign was a notable peak in Russia's positive health interventions, it was immediately undermined by the largest health crisis of the century—the arrival of the bubonic plague in Moscow. Following months of denial of its arrival, the state acted to respond only when the plague threatened its foreign trade. Most important, local physicians in Moscow credited the arrival of the cold as the solution to the plague, arguing that the climate could in fact defeat this dangerous threat. This incident marks the beginning of part 3, in which Russia's climatological and health challenges led its specialists to challenge, and even reject, established knowledge in Western Europe. This catastrophe undoubtedly contributed to a new focus on verifying the benefits or risks of Russia's climate for the health of its population in chapter 5. A new academy expedition, led by Dr. Peter Simon Pallas, reinvestigated the empire in a similar way to the Second Kamchatka Expedition decades earlier. Russia's physicians, including Dr. Matthew Guthrie, began to publish positive assessments of the Russians' ability to manage their health despite the endemic dangers of scurvy and syphilis, among others. By 1781, when Catherine sponsored the second major smallpox inoculation event, this time for her grandchildren, it appeared the Russian government had restored some of its progressive accomplishments despite the damage of the plague in 1771. Unfortunately, a global catarrh pandemic that began in Russia late in 1781 and overtook Europe and the Atlantic world in 1782 once again revealed Russia as a source of dangerous diseases in chapter 6. The label "Russian Catarrh" emerged from the idea that cold spaces like Russia generated cold diseases, particularly those affecting the lungs, such as catarrh. Guthrie would spend the next decade trying to prove that Russia's climate was not unhealthy, producing his "Dissertation on the Climate of Russia" (1790) as his final argument.[31] New scientific expeditions launched by the Russian Academy also gathered more evidence to prove that Russia's population could thrive in its environment, even suggesting that if there was a challenge it was in distant Kamchatka or the North Pacific islands.

At the dawn of the nineteenth century, therefore, the Russian scientific and medical establishment may have mitigated its disease burden, but Russia's foreign critics still held doubts. The Napoleonic invasion and the subsequent destruction of the Grand Armée obviously placed the European-wide discussion about Russia's climate and its dangers at the forefront of medical concerns. Much of the discussion after Napoleon's invasion was on uncovering Russian peasants' habits that allowed them to survive and thrive in a place so inhospitable to others, as Crichton had demonstrated. France's physicians tended to endorse the conclusion of Russia's eighteenth-century physicians, including Guthrie, but critics of Russia remained vocal. Crichton's work on consumption was even condemned as quackery.[32] Europe's perception of the positive improvements to health implemented across the previous century were quickly undone, not by the failure of the Russian government or its employees but rather by outside opinions. This should not undermine the accomplishments of the eighteenth century. In fact, it highlights how important it is to reclaim this narrative.

Part I

Structuring Knowledge

Chapter 1

Experiencing Climate, Observing People

The first English ambassador to Russia, Giles Fletcher, arrived in Moscow in 1588 to negotiate with the tsar's government for a reestablishment of English trade privileges. His negotiations failed, but he drew on his travels to publish a description of the empire, *Of the Russe Common Wealth*, in 1591. According to Fletcher, Russia's intemperate climate rendered much of the tsar's domains uninhabitable: "The countrie Northwards towards the parts of S. Nicolas and Cola, and Northeast towards Siberia, is all very barren, and full of desart woods by reason of the clymat, and extremitie of the cold in winter time."[1] This was not Fletcher's only reaction to Russia's climate, but the idea that Russia was dangerously cold, particularly in the northern stretch between Arkhangel'sk and Moscow, was a common idea across early-modern Europe.

European travelers in Fletcher's era shared his interest in the climate. Information about foreign lands was necessary to understand how one's body would react in a new environment. In the sixteenth century, Europeans accepted the principles of classical humoral theory. The idea of bodies composed of four humors (blood, phlegm, yellow bile, and black bile) that reflected four elements (air, water, fire, and earth) was common knowledge. Each humor had two characteristics: blood was hot and moist; phlegm was cold and moist; yellow bile was hot and dry;

black bile was cold and dry. Bodies had an internal balance of humors that defined a person's constitution. If blood was the dominant humor, the person was sanguine. If it was phlegm, the person was phlegmatic. Yellow bile produced choleric people, and black bile led to melancholic people. One's constitution, however, was not only defined by the internal composition of the humors but also by one's interactions with external influences (called the nonnaturals): air and climate; food and drink; activity and rest; retentions and evacuations; and sex. In general, people living in the same region would experience the same air and climate, likely consumed similar foods, and engaged in similar sorts of labor. Similar nonnatural conditions should produce similar sorts of bodies. If Russia was always colder than Fletcher's England, then its people were more likely to be phlegmatic or melancholic, which were the cold constitutions. Fletcher's observations were not only about climate and geography but also about Russia's population.

Fletcher was not the first European to visit Russia who remarked on the cold climate, nor would he be the last. As conditions deteriorated everywhere, the discussions only increased in frequency throughout the seventeenth century. The 1640s, in fact, was one of the coldest decades ever recorded, as the Little Ice Age reached a nadir, from a combination of global volcanic interruptions, low solar energy, and an unfortunate shift in oceanic currents. Decreasing food supplies produced ill health and epidemics, including one of the worst outbreaks of the bubonic plague in Europe since the fourteenth century.[2] European naturalists and physicians launched new investigations of the cold and the illnesses these conditions produced, particularly scurvy and rickets, as well as rheumatism and consumption. These men wrote to colleagues in Russia for advice on solving these problems produced by the cold. Robert Boyle investigated the properties of air in England, but turned to the tsar's physician in Moscow, Samuel Collins, for assistance. After all, who would know more about the cold than a physician working in Russia?

Physicians, naturalists, and diplomats living in Russia had different expectations about what the Russian Empire produced, both in terms of the bodies of its peoples and their health challenges. Samuel Collins, after leaving Russian service, capitalized on this growing interest when he published a narrative about life in the empire in 1667. His was the start of a new set of publications on Russia. These late seventeenth-century texts tended to challenge the idea that Russia was simply a cold space by documenting its hot and cold environments, and its varied peoples, who were often phlegmatic or melancholic, but who could be sanguine or choleric. These texts did not suggest the Russian Empire was a healthy region, as they agreed the climate was intemperate and diseases were widespread.

The Russian government was aware of the growing interest in Russia as a potential laboratory for European naturalists, and the pessimistic assessment of its conditions. The government, like other European countries, had always relied on its own diplomats and merchants to gather information about people, resources, geography, and climate, both inside its territory and within its neighbors'. By the end of the seventeenth century, Russia's diplomats began to publish travel narratives with this information following an important embassy trip to China in the 1690s, perhaps to counter the discussion of Russia's climate. The Russian government became a generator of knowledge, rather than serving as a foreign laboratory for experiments. This does not mean that the government successfully defeated the negative perceptions of the empire, but instead that the Russian government took its first steps to improve its fortunes. Russia at the dawn of the eighteenth century had set a new path for improving the health of its peoples and demonstrating its mastery of its climate.

Climate and Constitutions

In 1654, Cromwell's Commonwealth of England dispatched its first envoy to Russia, William Prideaux. Prideaux arrived in Arkhangel'sk to begin his overland trip to Moscow at an inauspicious time, as Russia was in the midst of an outbreak of the "contagious sicknesse" or, as we know it, the bubonic plague.[3] In Prideaux's first report on the current conditions, the situation was bleak: "The plague entered the city of Moscow as soon as the emperour was gone forth of it to the warrs, of which there hath dyed and been buryed by register taken upward of 200000, besides some thousands of bodies, that have had no other sepulchers than the bowels of dogs and hogs, that have eaten them, as well in the houses, as in the streets." The report went on: "This sickness hath passed (and is yet) in most places of this tract of the country for about 2000 miles in diameter, and now 'tis reported, that the kingdoms of Cazan and Astracan are also infected, and the mortality to be very great. Of those that dye the major part are men and children." Prideaux wrote to the English foreign secretary in hopes of receiving permission to remain in Vologda rather than proceed south to Moscow, as it "hath had less affliction by the sickness than any other in a great circuit thereabouts, here not having dyed past a thousand persons, and the most part of them poor people."[4] Without question, disease played an essential part in the relations among countries in the early-modern world.[5]

An educated, informed traveler in the seventeenth century, Prideaux's dispatches to London conveyed not only the information necessary for evaluating the success of his mission but also details for future English travelers to Russia how to navigate its distinct culture and unfamiliar climate. For centuries, educated Europeans knew that their health and well-being depended on residing in their native environment with their regular diet and activities. Deviating from the habits to which they were most accustomed could lead to their body becoming uneasy, if not diseased. The idea that the body was composed of four humors was unquestioned; these ideas had existed in Europe for more than a thousand years. For Prideaux to travel to a foreign climate and eat unfamiliar foods certainly would produce illness. To complete this trip in the middle of a pandemic only elevated the risks. In light of that knowledge, Prideaux's caution seems reasonable.

Reading Prideaux's correspondence about Russia with an eye toward its humoral language yields plentiful results. In his first letter when he wrote about the "contagious sicknesse," he also provided complete descriptions of the constitution (or humoral features) of the local population: "That, which hitherto I have observed (and learned of others) of this people, is, that the men are rather of a tall then middle stature; they are withal gross, and stronge; and those strangers, that deale with them, find them subtle and crafty, but are very pusillanimous. . . . 'Tis said, the men are much addicted and doe exercise the abominable sinne of sodomy with boyes, and use beasts; and in those vices not inferior to Turkes and Italians." His letter continued: "For the matter of victuals, both flesh and fish are here in great abundance, and good cheape. Their drinke is beer, mead (made of honey) that's good and pleasant. Both men and women of quality, that have meanes to spend, goe rich in their appariall, and weare many jewels, and in particular pearle in abundance; especially of those that are fisht in the Scottish sea, and are called by the name of Scottish pearle."[6]

Physical stature and descriptions of bodies, concern about sexual activity, and the quality of food served were all basic issues that future travelers would need to know. The mention that their accoutrements could be connected, albeit loosely, to Scotland suggested that a Scot might be a better choice for the position than an Englishman like

Prideaux. Neither the choice of topics nor the implication of other, better adapted, servitors had to be explained. Any literate person in the seventeenth century understood this descriptive language, both for its humoral and nonnatural implications.

Humoral theory was an interlocking, complex system of description, capable of explaining health and climate. The core of the system was a person's constitution (also characteristic or complexion), which was the balance of humors within an individual. Medical practitioners and the general public in the early-modern era understood that a sanguine person was strongly associated with blood (wet and hot), a phlegmatic person with phlegm (cold and wet), a choleric person with yellow bile (hot and dry), and a melancholic person with black bile (cold and dry). If the cold climate was the primary feature of the Russian Empire, then its residents were likely to be either phlegmatic or melancholic peoples. The historian Rebecca Earle has summarized phlegmatics as "prone to apathy" and melancholics as "prone to sadness."[7] An empire composed of sad, apathetic subjects may have been easy to rule, but it was unlikely to prosper as it lacked the industry, energy, and overall initiative of men and women from warmer climates.

Foreigners like Prideaux arrived in Russia with a belief that Russians had a fundamental weakness because their climate was colder than "temperate" Europe. Although geography and climate are not necessarily features of the body's humors (the naturals in Galenic terminology), both were key features of the nonnaturals, conditions outside the body that affected one's health. The nonnaturals were air and climate; food and drink; activity and rest; retentions and evacuations; and sex.[8] For a complete portrait of an individual, a bodily description would not be sufficient; one also needed to know what were the distinctive features of the climate, what type of foods were concerned, what type of work or leisure occupied the person, and what were their sexual preferences or how easily or not could they procreate.[9] Lifestyle descriptions could become quite lengthy, involving dress, skills, occupations, and even attitudes. Travel writers in the early-modern world provided endless details about the entire life cycle of peoples around the world, typically beginning with physical descriptions of an average man and woman, but then tracking the group from birth rituals to funeral practices. In the nineteenth century (and modern era), this type of narrative might be framed as an ethnography, especially if produced by a naturalist or a physician, but in the seventeenth century, the information provided was a complete humoral portrait, functioning as medical description.

Humoral theory was the medical system of the Greco-Roman-Islamic world for centuries, but it was also a system of rhetoric. Rhetoric, in this context, is "an organized, consistent coherent way of talking about practical discourse in any of its forms or modes," as the scholar Douglas Ehninger has defined.[10] Relying on a system of rhetoric enabled physicians, naturalists, and other educated elites to better convey significant information.[11] This information contributed to the so-called republic of letters—that is, the exchange of ideas among the literate elites of Europe in the early-modern era.[12] When Prideaux described Russia's conditions in 1654, he was confident that the foreign secretary in London would understand the connections to humoral idioms and its significance. Working within a defined system of rhetoric, however, also limited the potential exchanges into set patterns: Certain pieces of information had to be included. For seventeenth-century Russia, the diverse peoples of the empire would be described in similar terms, as a result of European expectations of this common climate, diet, and lifestyle.

Prideaux wrote as many observers would, describing the lives of Russians as if they were a uniform group, but most educated people of his time recognized individuals could have different constitutions, even in a similar environment. The fundamental importance of not only understanding the people and their bodies but also the climate, diet, and activities is the reason why these humoral descriptions saturate early-modern texts. If one had a diet primarily composed of phlegmatic foods from a cold and wet environment, like fish, then that person would be phlegmatic, in the same way that someone whose diet primarily consisted of red meat (blood) would more likely be sanguine. Someone born in a mountainous region, with its cold and dry air, would be understood to be melancholic. Mountain and melancholy were synonymous.

Differences could be revealed through illnesses. In the classical understanding of the humors, any illness was a sign that the humors had become unbalanced. A change in diet or climate produced disease, as any traveler could attest. All foods were converted to humors during digestion; having too much red meat, for example, produced too much blood, which might be made apparent if the patient had a fever or, as they understood it, an excess of heat. Changing climates was always linked to altering digestion, either too fast in heat or too slow in cold. In the former, the body might fail to absorb sufficient quantities of one humor; in the latter, "putrefaction," or the decay of material or humors inside the body, was possible. Both produced illnesses. Following this line of argument, removing excess humors to allow one's body to become naturally balanced was essential. Emetics or purgatives could be used to free the digestive system of potential putrefaction; bloodletting quickly solved excess heat in the body. By the early-modern era, anything consumable, whether chemical or herbal, might resolve an illness by offsetting the imbalance. If one had a fever, then white foods, which became phlegm, could be supplemented by rest to avoid heat or by cold baths to rebalance the body.

Any attempt to describe the humoral system at work in the seventeenth century is reductionist. It was a highly complex system with multiple factors influencing descriptions and treatments. Every physician believed their home environment was temperate and traveling anywhere beyond one's local environment risked ill health. A Scottish physician in Edinburgh would have a different conception of "temperate" than one from London, for example, not to mention those at work in southern France, northern Africa, or in the European colonies across the Atlantic. Prideaux was a diplomat and not a physician, but even he reflected the idea that Russia would be safer for a "northern" Scot than for a "southern" Englishman. Writing in the 1650s, Prideaux wrote with the confidence that Russia was a cold space.

Prideaux's conviction about Russia's climate was shared by naturalists. Robert Boyle, a fellow of the Royal Society of London, relied on information from Moscow for his analysis of cold air, which ultimately influenced what became known as Boyle's law on air pressure.[13] In 1665, he published *New Experiments and Observations Touching Cold*, which included examples drawn from texts written about Russia to document its "extreme degrees of Cold," which Boyle otherwise could not verify "in this temperate Climate of ours." To inform his view of Russia, Boyle relied on Russian travel records published in England, including those by Fletcher, in the sixteenth century. Many of Boyle's borrowed traveler anecdotes were incidents in which water froze extremely quickly, but he was also fascinated by incidents in which "the extreme Cold of Winter" made "gaping chinks" in the ground sufficient "that a childs head might well have been put into the cleft." Although it was not the central focus of Boyle's interest in the effects of cold on air pressure, he noted that these Russian visitors agreed that the climate was damaging to its people. Boyle quoted one merchant, a Captain James, who wrote that the cold "would be so extreme, that it was not endurable; no clothes were proof against it, no motion could resist it. It would moreover so freez the hair of our Eye-lids, that we could not see; and I verily believe, that it would have stifled a man in very few hours."[14]

Boyle's study only confirmed an English impression of Russia's innate coldness. He was not alone, as English physicians began to pursue cures for diseases thought to emerge from the cold in Russia. One of the earliest examples of this was the expectation that Russia's environment must have provided a solution for treating rickets, which was known to be caused by the cold and increasingly widespread by the end of the seventeenth century.

Nutritional diseases were fundamental problems in the early-modern world. Scurvy, beriberi, and rickets, among others, were seasonal diseases with devastating consequences, especially for children. Russians had some benefits in this arena. Rye bread, the traditional staple of the Russian diet, was rich in thiamin (vitamin B1), providing some protection against beriberi, which had reached epidemic status in Asia.[15] However, both scurvy (vitamin C deficiency) and rickets (vitamin D deficiency) were common. In an era before the discovery of vitamins, these diseases could be diagnosed only from their resulting symptoms rather than from an understanding of the underlying cause. Many cures that were proposed for either disease failed to address the vitamin deficiency, but if the patient's health improved, potentially from general improvements in diet, observers would reasonably assume that the treatment had addressed the disease.[16]

Rickets was first analyzed by English physician Dr. Francis Glisson, in his text *De rachitide* (1650), published the following year in London as *A Treatise of Rickets*. According to Glisson, rickets was a cold illness, the result of a "weak" (or cold-bodied) mother nursing her child to ill health.[17] The first Russian study of the disease would not be published until 1830, which identified it as the "English disease" for its notorious incidence rate in Britain.[18] It is possible that Russia's medical establishment considered rickets to be a foreign illness or a minor issue leading to this much later study; however, English physicians confronting a growing epidemic in the seventeenth century expected the coldest country in Europe to possess a local solution to this disease.

In 1694, another English physician, a Dr. Skinner, published the results of his investigation, that Russia did in fact naturally produce a treatment for rickets. It was a rare product from the Baltic Region: mannagrass seed. Mannagrass produces a small, edible seed; it grows naturally in northeastern Europe, from the Oder River at least as far east as Belorussia. The seed was harvested between May and July. Then the seeds were dried in the sun and finally were ground into a paste that could be used to produce a slightly sweet bread.[19] According to

Skinner, it was "a small white Seed that comes from Russia, by some called *Seed Manna,* I draw a Tincture, a Spirit and an Extract out of it, and give twenty Drops at a time in all the Childrens Meat and Drink." Skinner suggested it was preferable to the other options currently available, as the children "take it with Pleasure, because it's not ungrateful to the Pallat; Morning, Noon and Night, is often enough." According to Skinner, this mannaseed increased the body's ability to intake essential nutrients: "It opens Obstructions of the Liver and Spleen, strengthens the Brain and Spinal Marrow, and causeth a free Distribution of the Nourishments into all the Nervous Parts of the Body, whereby Nature becomes strong and vigorous, and the Spirits cheerful and lively."[20] Skinner's analysis is humoral; this tincture was capable of defeating the putrefaction of the liver and spleen that he believed caused rickets.

In the modern day, no one links nutritional diseases to putrefaction; however, in the early-modern world, most, if not all, cold diseases were the result of putrefaction. The idea that a cold environment like Russia both produced a disease and its treatment had long been an accepted part of humoral theory. It was logical for physicians to assume that if rickets was endemic to Russia, so too would a cure have been. Skinner's theory was sufficiently convincing that another English physician, Samuel Dale, included mannagrass seed in his pharmacopoeia published in 1705, describing *Gramen Mannae esculentum* as the "commonly called Manna-Grass or Russia Seed," and noting its "admirable virtues in the treatment of rickets."[21] Both the name "Russia Seed" and the idea that mannagrass seed could cure rickets began with Skinner a decade earlier, demonstrating that his idea circulated throughout the medical community. Decades later, British naturalists continued to recommend mannagrass seed as "a pleasant Food, proper for the Nourishment of Children and weak Persons," in hopes of encouraging domestic cultivation to limit Britain's dependence on Russia's exports.[22]

The optimism that Russia's environment produced a cure for rickets reflected a seventeenth-century idea: Russia's cold climate produced people with cold characteristics who suffered from (and ideally survived) cold diseases. This depiction was shared among diplomats and merchants working in Russia as well as by naturalists and physicians working outside the empire; the common idea uniting their discussion was humoral theory. This perception of Russia and its peoples had flaws, but Russia as a cold empire was not simply a negative assessment.

As the hope for a cure for rickets revealed, part of this idea was that Russia should be generating cures for cold diseases that could benefit other Europeans. Russia might have been cold, but it could also be productive.

Humoring Russia

When Prideaux observed the plague's damage to Russia in the early 1650s, the notion that Russia suffered from its cold climate was hardly new. Nor did Prideaux's time in the country convince him that Russia had a healthy environment. For others like Boyle or Skinner, Russia's coldness was an asset for the advancement of science, because it offered a climate that could not be matched elsewhere. Following Boyle's publication, new publications about life in Russia notably increased. In English, the first of these texts would arrive from Boyle's correspondent in Russia, the tsar's personal physician, Samuel Collins. The depiction of Russia, both the land and its people, was far more complicated for those who spent more time in the country. Collins was among the first to observe that Russia was not simply a cold climate but rather was an expansive empire with a complex social system. Its people were not only phlegmatic and melancholic but also exhibited an entire range of characteristics.

After returning to England, Collins published his well-known description of life in the country, *The Present State of Russia* (1667). Any physician describing a foreign land had to address the nonnaturals (i.e., air and climate; food and drink; activity and rest; retentions and evacuations; and sex). Accordingly, Collins's text included details on each. The contents would have been logical to Prideaux and Boyle, but Collins's view of the land and peoples reflected his eight years in Moscow. To him, Russian was two distinct spaces: one for the Russians that was warm and productive, and one for the non-Russian subjects that was cold and dangerous.

Collins's description of the Russians highlighted their unexpected warm features. This description is first found early in his text when he describes Russian children as "commonly strong and hardy," as opposed to weak, cold bodies. Even in Lent, the Russians "give themselves over to all manner of debauchery and luxury, and in the last week they drink as if they were never to drink more," all assessments of an active or hot people. The Russians also diligently observed multiple fasts every year, which should have sapped their strength and energy: "They eat no Fish, but feed on Cabbage and Cucumbers, and course Rye bread, and drink Canasse [kvass], which is a Liquor one degree below our small Beer."[23] Despite their diet and climate, the Russians remained healthy and strong.

Furthermore, Russians endorsed early marriage for their children, which again sat in opposition to the expectation of a typical cold person who should lack interest in sex and procreation, which were well-known as hot qualities. Without marriage to control the sexual impulses of Russians, their tendency would be for "Sodomy and Buggery, to which they are naturally inclined." Nor were sexual activities of Russians limited to men, as it was "but a venial Piccadillo for a Russ woman to prostitute her self to a Stranger, for they say her issue will be educated in the true ancient Faith." According to Collins, in having an active sex life, the Russians also struggled with venereal diseases, which were hot diseases, not well suited toward the climate. Venereal disease was a foreign acquisition, and therefore Russia and its people had no natural defenses nor solutions. As Collins summarized, "My Lady *Lues Venerea*. . . . gets into such a cold Countrey as this, she earths like a Badger so deep, that there's no driving of her out without a Pickaxe or Firebrand."[24]

Although Collins's Russians were active and strong, unusual for their climate, the other people of the empire were not. Collins described the Cherkassian "Tartars" as "a rude swarthy look'd people; their Women are very unhandsome, gross, and grossly given to drinking; so that at an Entertainment they will be drunk before meat comes on the Table, and with eating recover themselves, and after Dinner be drunk again, and then recover themselves by Dancing, which they love so much, that they count him a mean man who does not keep a Fidler in his house."[25] His characterization of them as "unhandsome, gross" indicates innate weakness and inability to control the passions (for alcohol, in this case), confirming a total lack of temperate qualities. When Collins described their type of government as "perfectly Anarchical," it underscored this assessment. In Collins's description, these Tatars were weak in body, and incapable of ruling themselves; in other words, they were cold. All of this was true despite their "Land" being "better and warmer" than the Russians, though it led them to be prone to excess, not control.

Siberia was a source of fascination for Collins, even though his account of the country relied on hearsay, having "spoken with one that was there." Its main feature was "so excessive cold . . . that water thrown up into the Air will descend congeal'd into Ice. The most Northern parts afford no Bread, but Fish in abundance, which they eat dryed instead of bread, and yet they live to a great age." Both the climate and the fish indicated that Siberia was populated by a cold people, which was confirmed by "no Beards but on their upper lip" on the men along the Chinese border.[26] Facial hair was one of the most visible signifiers of a hot (masculine) constitution.

Collins particularly identified the Samoyeds of northern Siberia as the more problematic of Siberia's peoples. The term *Samoyed* was part of the issue, as "Samogeda, or Tsamoeida, which signifies Canibals, or Men-eaters, for they eat those whom they conquer in battel." In a cold climate, with a diet of "most Fish," their cold constitution was inevitable. Therefore, "You can hardly distinguish the men and women by their visage, neither wear Beards, and both have faces like Baboons."[27] With the extreme conditions producing men who developed feminine qualities, Collins concluded that the Samoyeds were the least developed people in the empire, with little hope of future success.

Collins's text established a precedent for English-language descriptions of Russia. It was first printed in London in 1667 and reprinted three times in the next thirty years, indicating a high circulation. His imagery and descriptive language would appear in other narratives of Russia, and not necessarily as a direct borrowing but rather from a shared sense of the appropriate language to use to describe a foreign group. Jan Janszoon Struys was a Dutch sailor and later diplomat who spent two periods in Russia, the first in the tsar's service as part of an effort to develop a Caspian fleet in 1668 and the second as part of a Dutch diplomatic mission to Moscow in 1676.[28] His travel narrative was translated into multiple languages and circulated across Europe within two decades of his transit, including an English edition, *The Perilous and most Unhappy Voyages of John Struys* (1683). His arrival in the city of Pskov began with strong criticism of Russia's cuisine: "As for their Bread it is not much unlike our *New-castle* Coal for colour, but how it is of Tast I know no more than Man in the Moon, for neither my Appetite nor Curiosity could move me to it, Cabbage they have in great abundance, which is of a Tast like Sorrel, but close and white like ours, That and Cucumbers are the main ingredients whereof these People seem to be compounded, but more especially the latter, for *Cumber* attends them from the Womb to the Tomb, being held in perpetual Slavery by their Lords." He also discussed the climate, noting that "Moscou, and all the whole Countrey towards the North is capable of a very unwholsom Air, for those that are not brought up in it, being in the Winter exceedingly sharp and cold, and in the Summer hot and moyst." Although some might have expected the cold to be troubling, the heat of summer was no better: "It is there so hot in the Summer that a stranger cannot endure it, at what time also the Marshes and standing Pools so stink that one is ready to faint away: besides the great annoyance of Gnats, Muskettos and other Vermin, against which there is no way to defend ones Face."[29] Struys's Russia was not only extremely cold but also was extremely hot; either season made Russia's climate remarkably intemperate.

According to Struys, the extreme climate simply produced unbalanced people: "The Common people were formerly so irregular and void of Order that they would drink themselves full, and afterwards men and Women, setting aside all Reputation and Modesty commit sensual and beastly Actions together."[30] Struys's observations on the excessive sexual activity among Russians was only one more piece of evidence for him about the lack of a temperate climate and reasonable diet. Russia was a land of humoral unease.

The question implicit in Struys's description is how Russians functioned in spite of the persistent difficulties of the climate. To overcome the extreme cold, "In Winter they muffle up their Nose and Ears in Furs, especially when they go upon a Journey. And in Moscou it is well seen that may of the Inhabitants have neither Nose nor Ear, which they say is by coming out of the bitter cold Air into a hot Stove." In summer, Russians could eat fruit, most of which held cold and moist attributes, to offset the heat: "The Fruits they have are Pears, Apples, Quince, Medlars, Cherries Plumbs, and of these several kinds." This did not produce a land perfect in balance, as excess both in terms of Russians' sexual habits as well as their fondness for alcohol led to a variety of obstacles, but the state could intervene when necessary: "This great Disorder was lately remedied by the care of the Czar, who, by the advice of the Patriarch, put down all the small Tap-houses throughout the whole Empire, appointing in every Town and Village one public House, or Kaback, which they are to farm of the Emperour himself."[31]

Struys's colorful observations on Russians' lifestyle only confirmed the imagery and ideas already circulating from Collins's narrative. Struys was not a trained physician like Collins, but his descriptions operated along similar lines, because both relied on humoral tropes to depict a foreign land. Nor were these ideas limited to physicians and diplomats. Philippe Avril was a French Jesuit who became an Asian explorer. He traveled for six years through the Caucasus and Middle East, and spent time in Russia, traveling between Astrakhan and Moscow. After leaving Russia, he also wrote a travel narrative that was translated and published in English in 1693. Although the tsar denied permission for the Jesuits to travel from Moscow across Siberia to China, Avril took the opportunity to discuss the empire with the merchants in Moscow's markets. After being introduced to so-called Chinese merchants "though they were only Tartars, gave us great insight in to both Countries [Siberia and China], which had been but so obscurely known till very lately; and in regard they Traffick as well with the Chineses as with the Muscovites, and for that they had been both at Pekin and Moscow, both Roads were known alike to them."[32] Following this conversation, Avril detailed six routes crossing from Moscow to China, most traveling through Siberian cities but some moving through Central Asia, listing towns, peoples, and challenges for each route. Without tsarist permission to travel, these were only Avril's expectations, not his firsthand observations.

Avril, however, still had his personal experiences of moving through European Russia from Astrakhan to Moscow along the Volga River. As was the case with so many Europeans, Avril's interest was focused on the extreme climate. Leaving Astrakhan, for example, he wrote: "We began to feel the approach of Winter, and the difference of the Climate, of which the Artick Pole, toward which we were insensibly advancing, made us sensible in spite of our Teeth. And in regard we had not so well fortifi'd our selves, as we ought to have done before our departure from Astrakhan against the Cold, . . . we thought we should have been frozen to Death." Avril noted the dichotomy of Russia's extreme conditions: "A North Wind, no less sharpe and cutting, then violent and boisterous arose, and in a little time stop'd the Course of the Volga, by freezing up the River" that "reduc'd me to a very low Condition of Body for want of good looking after," but the resulting "extremely serene and clear" winter days eased the work for merchant caravans that found it easier to transport goods along the frozen river.[33]

And if the winter was not sufficiently a challenge, Avril also raised concerns about the summer: "The Summer heats are not to be endured in that place; insomuch that the people are oblig'd to bath several times a day." Aside from the difficulty of balancing one's humors in the extreme climate, the locality produced food that was inherently risky. "The Soils bears all sorts of Fruits, and in great abundance; nor does their deliciousness give way to the plenty. More especially their Melons are remarkable for their most exquisite taste; and it is as rare a thing to meet with a bad or a willowish Melon there, as it is unusual to find a good one in France."[34] Although it is clear that Avril enjoyed Astrakhan's melons, Europeans had been involved for more than a century in a debate about whether too much fruit was dangerous for a European body. This was a recurring fear in the ongoing settlement in the Americas.[35] The fact that part of Russia had a similarly balmy climate brought the same tropical risks for Europeans.

Beyond his personal observations, Avril relied on the secondhand information gathered in the markets of Astrakhan and Moscow from traveling merchants to provide insight into the people and climate of Russia's Asian territories. He identified his best informants as Tatars, but that label could have applied to any number of Turkic and Central Asian peoples, including Tatars from Kazan' and Siberia. Therefore, as a source for the people of Siberia, risks were associated with Avril's reliability, but given the relative dearth of information about this enormous territory, even the secondhand information he provided could be useful. He described "Siberians" as a diverse group, as "others who are called Ostiaki, Bratski, Jacuti, and Tongusi, who are scatter'd all along the Lakes and Rivers that lye between Siberia and the Country of the Monguls. But in regard they have all the same Physiognomy, and use the same Language as the Calmoucs, 'tis very probable that they are only some separated *Hordes*, that having been domesticated by degrees, by conversation with the *Muscovites*, at length became subject to their Dominion."[36]

In Avril's assessment, the potential of the government to transform the inhabitants of Siberia into productive subjects was limited: "They are all swarthy complexion'd, but more inclining to Olive-Colour than Black. Their faces are usually broad, falling in below, and jutting out above; their eyes are small, but sparkling and full of fire; their noses short and very flat, with little hair either upon their upper Lips, or Chins: Their Status somewhat about the common size, well set, and clean limb'd, with an Air stern and resolute, without any thing of Cruelty or Savageness."[37] Their "Olive-Colour" complexion suggested a choleric or melancholic disposition, but the lack of facial hair confirmed a cold body. The lack of "Cruelty or Savageness" made these groups better potential subjects than any that were violent or warlike (hot, in other words), but their lifestyle (i.e., the connection to the Russians), could transform the bodies only so far.

Although Avril drew on his personal experiences in European Russia and access to merchants to provide a more complete portrait of the

Russian Empire, he also reacted to earlier narratives about the country. He criticized Struys for incorrectly positioning Astrakhan as fifty leagues from the mouth of the Volga River, when it was only thirteen. Avril also drew distinctions between his travels along the Volga and that of the diplomat Adam Olearius, who moved along the river more than five decades earlier.[38] Collins, Struys, and Avril may not have agreed on Russia's conditions, but they were part of a broader conversation about Russia's people and climate. The similarity of their depictions and the association with humoral principles is all the more likely because these men read the earlier narratives.

By the end of the seventeenth century, multiple narratives about Russia circulated throughout Europe. The most detailed of these were produced by those men who lived and traveled in Russia, but others still aspired to write about Russia without firsthand experience. This was the case for Jodocus Crull, in his *Account of the Antient and Present State of Muscovy*, published in London in 1698. Crull was born in Hamburg, received his medical doctorate from the University of Leiden in 1679, and was appointed as a fellow of the Royal Society in London two years later.[39] Throughout his text, he included similar details to Collins's work, citing the same events, people, and diseases, but in greater detail at many points, despite not having Collins's long career in Russia.

Unsurprisingly, the two physicians shared an interest in relating the people, climate, food, customs, and habits. Crull began his text with a sweeping declaration of Russia's climate as the most important feature of the country. Russia "is generally excessive Cold in the Winter, and the Heats in the Summer, during the space of two or three Months, very intense and violent. The Country is generally flat and Sandy, full of Trees and Woods, so that Muscovy, in a manner, appears to be one continual Forest." Crull, however, also suggested that the cold climate was actually an asset for the Russians' development: "The Muscovites are from their Infancy inur'd to all sorts of Hardship, their Children being seldom suckled above two or three Months; and this with the coldness of their Climate, and their sparing Diet, makes them very fit to endure the Fatigues of War, being especially very resolute in defending of Places; which they will maintain to the utmost extremity."[40]

With the cold climate producing a positive benefit, Crull was optimistic about the qualities of Russian men and women. "The Muscovites are of a middle Seize as to their Stature, strong proportioned, of the same colour as the other Europeans in the Northern Parts. But they much affect Corpulency, especially among Persons of Quality. Long Beards, and great Mustachios are in great request among them, which they look upon as tokens of Virility." Russian women were also positively described, "of a middling Stature, neither too tall nor too little, and generally well proportion'd before they are married, but after they have had several Children, inclining to Fatness." Agreeing with Collins, Crull noted the Russians' propensity to drink excessively: "From hence also proceed these frequent Irregularities, Disorders and Excesses in Debaucheries, even to sin against the Course of Nature, not only with Men, but also with Beasts." In spite of the criticism, however, Crull was generally positive about their characteristics: "The Muscovites are a People of great Wit, Cunning and Dexterity, not wanting Ingenuity in anything they undertake, as has been sufficiently experienced by those, who have had Opportunity to deal with them, either by way of Commerce or otherwise."[41]

Crull's characterization only confirmed the Russians were a humoral enigma. The cold climate should have produced a people that were prone toward inactivity, and yet Crull and Collins believed the Russians were active and hardy. Crull suggested one solution to this issue: The Russians reliance on their *banias* (bathhouses), with their exposure to extreme heat. "These Baths are the universal Remedies of the Muscovites, not only for cleansing their Bodies, but also for the Preservation of their Health, which being thus from their Infancy inur'd to the greatest Extremities of Heat and Cold, makes them to be of a very strong and healthy Constitution, and for the generality long liv'd," For Crull, the only challenge to their health was the recent introduction of venereal diseases from Poland, where the Russians "made a very intimate Acquaintance with the Venereal Disease, which, in so cold a Climate as theirs, sticks very close to them."[42] Crull's assessment of venereal disease in Russia borrows directly from Collins's text, but his interest in the role of the bania demonstrates his willingness to move beyond Collins's initial assessment.

Compared with the Russians, the other peoples of the empire did not fare as well. The Finno-Ugric Maris along the Volga River, for example, "are a Nation barbarous, treacherous and cruel, living upon Robbery, and addicted to Sorcery." Furthermore, "Polygamy is used among them, even so as to Marry two or three Sisters at a Time." Both features revealed a people whose habits only demonstrated excess, or an imbalance in the humors.[43] It could be the lack of the habit of the steam bath left their bodies ill-suited toward their local environs.

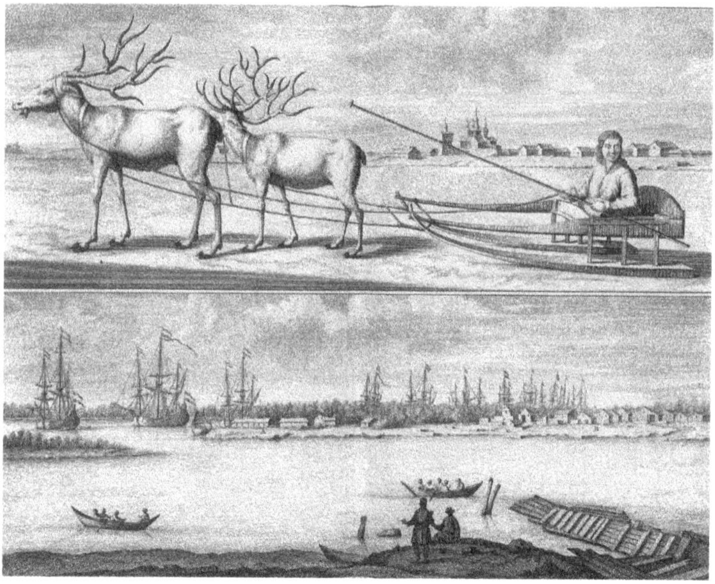

Figure 1.1. This image, which was included in a Dutch merchant's account of traveling through Moscow to South Asia, highlights the Samoyeds connection to the cold north with their reindeer sleigh. Image from Cornelis de Bruijn, *Reizen over Moskovie, door Persie en Indie* (1714). "Samojeedse slede met hare Rendieren; Scheepsbouwery of werf buiten Archangel," Rare Book Division, The New York Public Library, New York Public Library Digital Collections, accessed June 9, 2024, https://digitalcollections.nypl.org/items/510d47e1-cdfa-a3d9-e040-e00a18064a99.

Russia's port on the Caspian Sea, Astrakhan, was populated by Tatars, who "are of an ill shape, low and fat, with large Faces, and little Eyes, of an Olive colour, full of wrinkles in their Faces, they wear little Beards, and keep their Heads shaved; but the Women are much handsomer." This lack of facial hair (i.e., the "little Beards") was long known as a sign of men with a colder nature. The "olive" color of their skin, however, suggested the other warm-blooded people of the Mediterranean. The Tatars' confused characteristics may have been linked to the opposing extremes in the environment: "The Climate in those Parts is very hot, the Heats in the Months of September and October much exceeding our Dog-days; notwithstanding which, the Winter, which seldom exceeds two Months here, is so cold, that this large River is commonly frozen up, and bears Sledges" (figure 1.1).[44]

Crull had an easier time describing the people of the empire whose residence was in the far north, which he believed lacked the experience of the extreme heat that troubled the people of the south. The Samoyeds, for example, garnered a lengthy depiction in his book. Their climate and diet were inextricably linked: "The length of the Winter Season making their Ground not fit for Tillage, they have no Corn nor Cattle, so that they are contented, to live upon what Nature affords them; their Food being Fish dry'd in the Wind and Sun, instead of Bread, Honey and Venison."[45] Fish primarily had a cold, moist characteristic, producing excess phlegm in the body; people subsisting on a fish diet were likely phlegmatic. The physical description of the Samoyeds confirmed this diagnosis: "Their Stature is very low and mean, having very short Legs, . . . their faces large and flat without Beards, and their Eyes very little, like the Tartars, but not so sparkling. The Women here are very ugly, so that by their Faces and Cloaths; which are exactly like to the Men's, their Sex is not to be distinguished at first fight." Short men, with an absence of facial hair, were clearly marked as cold figures. The lack of distinct sexual features between men and women drew a portrait of an appropriately sexless community, as cold men lacked interest in procreation. Despite this, Crull noted with surprise that Samoyed men "are very jealous of them [women], being extreamely nice in preserving their Wives for their own use."[46] How Crull managed to comment on the sex lives of the Samoyeds without having any practical experience raises some valid questions about his observations on their sexual morality.

Although the conclusion of Collins, Struys, Avril, and Crull might have differed, without question, a humoral knowledge influenced their assessments of the bodies of the Russian Empire. The concern about the extreme climate and the negative consequences for its subject posed a clear obstacle for the Russian Empire. Whereas the men who worked for Russia, like Collins, observed some positive features at least for the Russians, the views of short-term visitors and foreigners who never entered the country tended to be negative. By the end of the seventeenth century, if the Russian government wanted to confront these pessimistic assessments, a more active publishing effort, driven by its employees, could shift the conversation.

A Healthy Empire?

There was not a European consensus about the nature of Russia's climate nor a single view of the types of bodies of its subjects. Collins may have been considered more knowledgeable based on his years in Moscow and service to the tsar, but he was not the only author commenting on Russia's conditions, much less the only physician to comment on the health of imperial subjects. By the end of the century, the idea that Russia was simply a cold climate with an unhealthy environment tended to dominate European assessments of the empire. When the eighteenth century began, the Russian government became more active in gathering and publishing information, thus sponsoring a narrative to combat the more sensational accounts of the cold that had become common.

The frequency of complaints about the extreme cold in travel narratives turned the experience of cold into an expected feature of any record of life in Russia. In 1697, for example, Thomas Allison, a captain for one of the ships of the Russia Company operating out of Arkhangel'sk, published a day-by-day log of the transit from Russia to England to explain his unfortunate wintering off the coast of Russia. Aside from the struggle of managing to secure sufficient supplies of food and fuel for fires, the crew struggled with frostbite and scurvy, other well-known cold illnesses.[47] Publishing the tale of survival in London two years later only added more evidence of Russia's unsafe climate.

Those who found Russia's conditions manageable were also there, but their records often remained unpublished, perhaps because their experiences in Russia did not conform to the expectations of readers back in the West. Another Russia Company captain, William Baker, for example, kept his own log of a voyage to Arkhangel'sk in 1702, only three years after Allison's cautionary tale was published. The merchants arrived in the summer and departed Arkangel'sk before the harbor froze in the fall. On this particular voyage, Baker arrived in September, unloaded his cargo over the course of a week, despite the challenge navigating the harbor in "fresh gales of rain." He then supervised the provisioning of the boat for the return trip, loaded the exports from Arkhangel'sk, and departed in October without incident. It did snow on more than one day during the process, but this only served as an opportunity for Baker to enjoy the hospitality of the other English merchants living in the city, mentioning that "Mr. Pendlke and Mr. Lloyd made [him] very welcome."[48] If Allison's text was a cautionary tale of the dangers of Russia's cold climate, Baker's notes demonstrate that it still was possible to thrive in these conditions, much like the Russians had obviously done.

Like other European powers, the Russian government had always relied on its diplomats to investigate its neighbors and trade partners; diplomatic missions to the Middle East or Central Asia had long been avenues for gathering information.[49] The attempt to open direct contact with China in the middle of the seventeenth century would do no less. The state commissioned a Bukharan merchant, Seitkul Ablin, to gather information on the China trade. Ablin's information provided data for the first official embassy led by Fedor Isakovich Baikov in 1653, and Ablin's return trips to China eventually informed the second embassy led by Nikolai Spafarii in 1675.[50] The reports from these expeditions and embassies were kept in Moscow and were not prepared for publication in Russia or abroad. Even political exiles in Siberia in this period, like Iurii Kirzhanich, generated reports of the people of Siberia, but their assessments remained protected information.[51] Even as foreigners who had visited Russia published narratives about life in the country, Russians did not. Although former employees like Collins did publish when they left Russia for Europe, the Russian government was more invested in protecting information than in sharing it with a literate audience.

With publications such as Crull's or Allison's offering cautionary tales, Russia began to capitalize on its embassies as a source of information. In 1692, Tsar Peter I Alekseevich (r. 1682–1725) appointed a foreign diplomat, Eberhard Isbrand Ides, to act as his ambassador to China and appointed Adam Brand from Lubeck as the embassy's secretary.[52] The embassy included more than 250 men, including nobles and merchants, both to negotiate new terms following Nerchinsk as well as to investigate the market in Beijing, "where Silk, Cloath, Gold and Silver, Jewels and all sorts of fine Manufactures, were sold." Ides also toured "the Emperor's Dispensary, which I was willing to make some Scrutiny into, it being full stock'd with all sorts of Roots, Herbs, and Med'cines."[53] Ides had no formal medical training, but clearly had an interest, which was typical for merchants and diplomats in the early-modern era (figure 1.2).

Both Ides and Brand relied on the same humoral rhetoric in their narratives as their predecessors. Therefore, not all of their observations were positive. Outside of Tobol'sk, for example, Brand described the Ostiaks as "low of Stature, and very deformed; besides which, both Men and Women constantly are subject to a certain Weakness in their Eyes, the cause of which they attribute to a want of Bread; which being a scarce Commodity among them, they seldom are masters of it, unless they are by chance furnish'd with it by Travellers; which happening very rarely in so remote a Country, we supplied what we were able to spare; and instead of Bread, they make use of the same Fish dried."[54] On the banks of the Ob River, Ides described the Ostiaks as "a poor

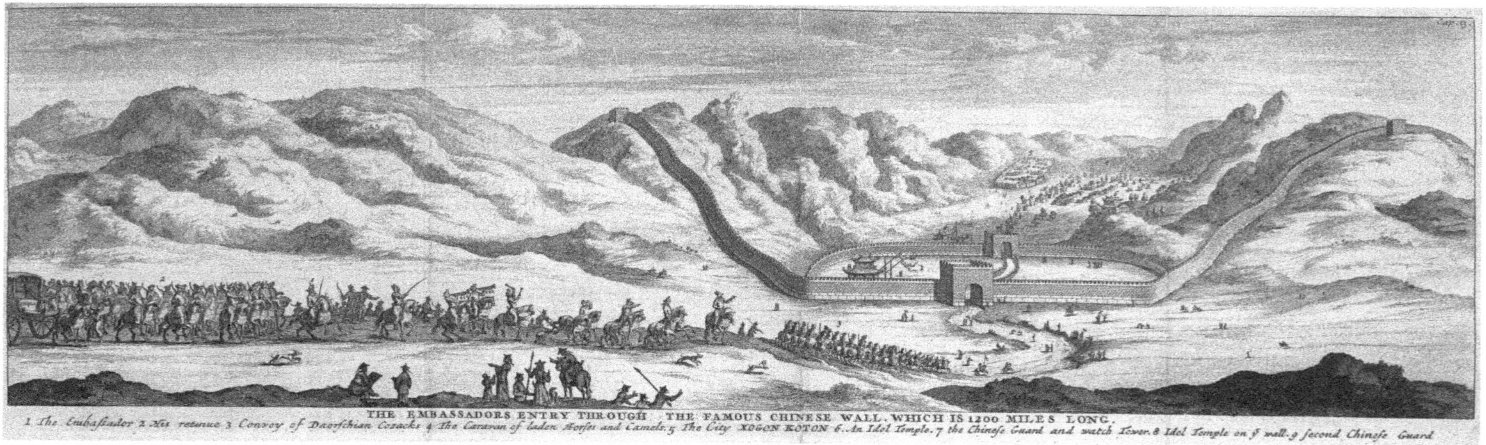

FIGURE 1.2. This panorama depicts the arrival of Ides's embassy at the border. The embassy travels through unsettled Siberia territory, while the Chinese side of the border depicts several communities. "The Embassadors entry through the famous Chinese wall which is 1200 miles long," General Research Division, New York Public Library Digital Collections, accessed June 9, 2024, https://digitalcollections.nypl.org/items/510d47e2-5bc0-a3d9-e040-e00a18064a99.

People, and live very miserable in sorry Hutts. . . . They are all of a middle Stature, most of them Yellowish or Red haired; and their Faces and Noses disagreeably broad; they are weak and unable to labour hard, not at all enclined to Warrs, and utterly uncapable of Military Exercises."[55] Ides was very clear that with a diet composed entirely of phlegm-induced fish, these cold men were weak and passive.

Brand drew attention to the persistent problem of the cold climate, following in the long tradition of Europeans complaining about the empire's extreme conditions. Nearing Nerchinsk among the Tungus, for example, the climate "proved very troublesome to us by reason of the Coldness of the Weather, which was so excessive, that our Victuals and Drink (which was only fair Water) froze, and turn'd to Ice, before we could bring it from hand to mouth."[56] As for the Tungus peoples, "they were formerly a War-like Nation, governed by its own Princes, inhabiting a very large Countrey" until they were conquered by the Russians.[57] What Brand failed to mention, and may not have known, is that the Tungus had not been conquered but rather defected from China to the Russian side of the border for better treatment.[58] "As to their Persons, they are very lusty and well proportion'd, their Cloaths being nothing but the Skins of Beasts, with the Furrs on the outside of divers Colours, neither Sex being distinguish'd by the least difference in their Habits." In other words, the Tungus were a contradiction. A warlike people implied a hot constitution, but the climate suggested otherwise. Brand, however, was certain he had discovered their secret: "For no sooner are their Children come into the World, but they lay them in the Summer in cold Water, in the Winter in the Snow; by which means they are so accustomed to Cold, that they are the hardiest People in the World," providing them sufficient strength "to defend themselves against the Violence of the Cold." Most important, this extreme weather training not only prepared Tungus men for their warlike futures but also provided sufficient heat that these men ardently pursued sex, as "all of them have several Wives," whereas people with a cold constitution were more likely to be disinterested in sexuality and procreation.[59]

Discussing the ability of the Tungus to overcome the quality of the climate implicitly criticized the Ostiaks, who had let the climate and diet define their characteristics. As a result, one group was active, sexual, and potentially aggressive, whereas the other was indolent and passive. In terms of managing Siberia, the Ostiaks should have been easy to control, whereas the Tungus would need more active intervention.

The humoral composition of each people made this apparent to anyone reading Brand's or Ides's narrative. As accounts from a state-sponsored embassy, both Brand and Ides could be viewed as the response to Collins, Struys, or Avril. Although each offered criticism of imperial subjects, the story of the Tungus indicated that Siberians could overcome their environment as the Russians did. It was not that all of the imperial subjects were intrinsically weaker from the climate or diet; the nonnaturals could be overcome if the people were willing to take the necessary steps to harden their bodies for these extreme conditions.

Although the embassy was an official undertaking, it did not guarantee access to each community across the entire empire. Brand recorded one incident in which he paid an Ostiak village for access to the interiors of their homes, with a "small Present of Bread and Salt to the Owners." Brand did not mention any difficulty communicating with the Ostiaks, but was confident that he had purchased an all- access pass to every part of the village: "One among them, somewhat bigger than the rest, and distinguish'd by certain Figures, invited my Curiosity to take a full View of it. Being entred, I found three Women lying upon the Ground, who at the sight of me arose from their places, and by their noddings and threatenings sufficiently testified their displeasure of seeing a Stranger interrupt them in their retirement; but being sensible that I had prepared my way by the Presents given to the Owners, I took, notwithstanding all their wry Faces, the liberty to search every corner of the Hutt."[60] Brand seemed to lack any concern with intruding on sleeping women and then investigating every corner of the residence. Instead, he was quite confident that his small presents guaranteed his rights. This would one of the first such instances recorded by Europeans traveling through Siberia, but it would not be the last.[61]

Brand's casual disregard for the feelings of these women was certainly part of the expectation that Russia and its government officials could treat imperial subjects as objects of scientific inquiry. Their participation may have been necessary to gain access, or act as a translator to explain local customs, habits, or religious traditions, but only in a subservient role. Even an embassy official, such as Ides, did not treat Russia's subjects any more humanely than the others. Gaining access to Siberia may have produced firsthand accounts of the subjects of the empire, but this process provided no more respect for the people under observation than did the men who never left Moscow.

When Ides and Brand published their accounts, neither man rejected the assessments of earlier writers. In fact, at times, their accounts confirmed some of the earlier humoral stereotypes. They also demonstrated, however, a path to challenge the representations of Russia's climate and population being published by those outside its borders. When the Russian government created the Academy of Sciences in the 1720s, it was an official decision to generate information about the empire. If diplomats failed to refute negative depictions of the empire, perhaps physicians and naturalists working for the state could succeed?

Chapter 2

Training Physicians, Exchanging Information

Medicine in eighteenth-century Russia reflected the wide variety of ideas and nosological classification schemes in place across Europe. Physicians and natural scientists, as well as the educated elite, had a working knowledge of Hippocratic-Galenic medicine. It informed a system of rhetoric at work in the seventeenth and eighteenth centuries, as humoralism and its conception of a body's constitution became the basis for understanding foreign places and people. At the same time, although these particular concepts had become commonplace, medical knowledge evolved beyond its Galenic foundations. Practicing humoralists preferred treatments that expelled excess humors to restore a natural balance with bloodlettings, emetics, and purgatives, whereas other practitioners preferred adding new substances (*materia medica*) into the body as an alternative to, or in combination with, expelling the excess. This change in therapeutics was based on improvements in the study of anatomy, chemistry, and botany, among other fields of science, that had fostered new ideas about the body during the seventeenth century.[1] These advancements in the natural sciences improved medicine. Herman Boerhaave, the most famous physician in early eighteenth-century Europe, made important contributions to botany to establish his reputation, but he had been trained broadly, including in chemistry and anatomy. His training reflected a generational shift in the way physicians were educated. Humoral language had not fallen out of use, but its value as a medical description was only one tool in a practitioner's therapeutic bag.

The improvements in science contributed to a diversification of medical practice by the beginning of the eighteenth century. Iatrophysics posited the origins of health and disease in the anatomical (physical) actions of the body. Iatrochemistry argued that the chemical balance inside the body was the key. Both theories were evolutions of humoral thought, but careers could be made by adhering to one theory over another. In practice, however, treatments might have been quite similar, as the entire practice of medicine remained embedded in trial-and-error experiments and grounded in a humoral understanding of the body's composition. In the eighteenth century, physicians were trained in all these disciplines. Unlike for their predecessors, training in chemistry and botany was essential for physicians to prescribe drugs, and some work either in the anatomy theater or even in a hospital was thought to be an asset in assessing patients. Medical knowledge based on traditional texts like Galen's or Avicenna's became only a part of a spectrum of information, produced by a conversation between practitioners on one side and natural scientists and an educated public on the other.

The conception of the bodies of Russia's subjects reflected these changing medical theories as well as ongoing fieldwork of physicians and naturalists in the empire. Physicians and naturalists both adopted the eighteenth century's interest in classification systems. The Russian Empire was almost *terra incognita*; ample space to study and analyze new animals, plants, and people. All these men wanted to discover how the people of the empire adapted to its distinct climate and geography. As important was the question of whether Russians could settle and occupy the empire's extensive territories. This was a question all of Europe confronted. For European settler colonialism to continue, solutions for assuring healthy bodies in diverse climates needed to be found, not only in tropical conditions in the Caribbean or Indian Ocean but also in cold places like Russia.[2]

Therefore, who led the process to explore, document, and classify the peoples, plants, and minerals of the empire was an increasingly central question. Would this discussion be led by men chosen by the Russian government or by visitors without attachment to the state? Would their observations highlight Russia's successes or reveal its inability to master Eurasia? The discussion occurring among physicians and naturalists was not a disinterested scientific pursuit but rather an ongoing, and potential critical, assessment of Russia's governing strategies. Unfortunately for the Russian Empire, this discussion was not easily controlled through official channels or by state employees. Humoral concepts, after all, were in general use among Europe's educated population, any of whom could become a new critic of Eurasia's largest empire.

Boerhaave's Curriculum

The key figure for Russia's medical future was Herman Boerhaave, a professor at the University of Leiden's medical school. Of the physicians employed by the Russian state, the overwhelming majority were either trained at Leiden or at the programs established by students of Boerhaave in Göttingen, Jena, and Edinburgh, among others. Boerhaave's innovative curriculum at Leiden, therefore, was the core of Russia's medical education throughout the eighteenth century. Even once its influence began to wane as new ideas emerged, the paths to Russian employment from these universities remained. The principles of Boerhaave's curriculum were embedded in medical practice throughout the empire.

In the seventeenth century and earlier, physicians were educated as a separate profession from surgeons and apothecaries. There were far more of the latter group than the former at work in the empire.[3] Although physicians held a university degree (doctor of medicine, MD), surgeons and apothecaries were skilled tradesmen who learned their craft after years of apprenticeships. Physicians also worked as apprentices, but the university degree remained a marker of distinction between the two groups. Before Boerhaave, as the historian of medicine G. A. Lindeboom observed, "Surgery was still a discipline not taught in many universities and often practised by illiterates, who did not understand Latin, the language of science, and who were often despised by the learned physicians."[4] The absence of surgery in a curriculum based on humoral precepts is logical. Rebalancing the humors within the patient did not take the physical manipulation of the body, but rather adjusting the nonnaturals (i.e., food, climate, activity, rest) to restore the original composition of the patient.[5] Therefore, the inclusion of anatomy and practical experience, including training in surgery and work with patients in a hospital, in the medical curriculum at Leiden was a major innovation to the study of medicine. This change reflected the arguments of the iatrophysical school, focusing on the physical body. In the modern era, this idea seems patently obvious, but at the dawn of the eighteenth century, it was groundbreaking.

On the one hand, this change might have been a surprise. Boerhaave's predecessor in the chair of medicine at Leiden, Franciscus Slyvius, was one of the leading figures of the iatrochemical school.[6] He was responsible for the construction of a new chemical laboratory in Leiden, and its inclusion in the curriculum. On the other hand, adopting both iatrochemistry and iatrophysical ideas was not the end of the innovations. Boerhaave began his career in Leiden as the head of the new botanical gardens, the study of which also entered the curriculum as some training in *materia medica* became essential to treat patients. With the Netherlands sitting in the center of a global empire, the new gardens at Leiden had plant specimens gathered from all corners of the Dutch reach.[7] Rather than posit medicine as the study of a science with its foundation in classical knowledge, by the end of the seventeenth century, Boerhaave and his colleagues at Leiden had created a distinct curriculum that incorporated elements from all of the new ideas produced by natural scientists.

In the first two decades of the eighteenth century, Leiden's reputation positioned it at the pinnacle of medical schools in Europe. The curriculum it developed was based in the instruction of all medical sciences first, and then it expanded to include clinical teaching in an instructional hospital. It covered the traditional knowledge of the humors as well as recent innovations in chemistry, physics, and botany to produce a new kind of physician.[8] It broke all traditions with the past by expecting physicians to have treated patients in person. This aspect of the curriculum reflected Boerhaave's respect for the work of the English physician Thomas Sydenham, who developed a new field of medicine known as nosology, or the categorization of diseases by symptoms.[9] Although Sydenham did not emphasize the study of anatomy, or the reliance on traditional humoral remedies such as bloodletting and purgatives, his nosologic system emerged from observation, an experience that required clinical practice.[10]

By the late seventeenth century, nosology had emerged as a practical solution to a growing problem in medical theory. Endemic diseases situated within a community proved humoral logic; people experiencing the same places, food, and climate should experience similar physical reactions. Epidemics and pandemics, however, were difficult to diagnose and treat through traditional humoral medicine. Each patient had his or her own constitution, which reflected their personal balance of the humors and could be altered by food, the environment, or physical activity. But the question of how to explain the plague, consumption, or dysentery, which acted on large groups with different constitutions, and, as Sydenham argued, were connected to seasons and the climate remained unanswered. Humoralists might look to one nonnatural as a common cause—for example, spoiled grain might be experienced by an entire community causing a disease outbreak. As more epidemics were recorded covering greater territory and different environments, those likely causes seemed less probable. Criticism of the traditional system had led to other ideas about transmission vectors. By the beginning of the eighteenth century, certain diseases, including "syphilis, inflamed eyes, and the itch, and, less often, consumption, plague, and dysentery" were understood to be contagious, in other words, moving from person to person rather than caused by a humoral imbalance condition.[11] Teaching diseases from a nosological approach, however, allowed physicians to disagree on the cause of disease but agree on the symptoms and potential treatments.

Boerhaave did not reject any of the competing medical theories of the time, rather he developed a curriculum that could embrace humoralism, iatrophysics, iatrochemistry, and nosology to train physicians in practical applications of this knowledge. At Leiden, students listened to lectures, but they also worked in the chemical laboratory, the botanical garden, the anatomy theater, and even in the school's hospital treating patients. More than one historian has argued this diversity in disciplines was why Leiden became the leading medical school for students across Europe in the first half of the eighteenth century.[12] It was remarkably progressive and marked a significant break from the medical and scientific education of the previous century. Borrowing ideas from multiple medical theories was a practical solution to the growing issue of public health, but Leiden became the institution that formalized this catchall system for Europe.[13]

Boerhaave's accomplishments led him to become one of the leading figures of Europe in the first quarter of the century. He was sufficiently well known that Tsar Peter I Alekseevich (r. 1682–1725) visited Leiden to meet Boerhaave and tour the university on his second embassy to Europe. According to the Dutch journals *Europische Mercurius* and the *Amsterdame Courant*, Peter arrived in Leiden on March 28, 1717, and arranged to meet Boerhaave the following morning. Boerhaave gave the tsar a personal tour of the University of Leiden's library, its anatomy theater, and the botanical garden.[14]

Boerhaave's reputation extended well beyond his meetings with Europe's monarchs. His students established new medical schools across Europe, including in Göttingen and Jena, among other schools in Germany.[15] Practical instruction alongside medical theory became the basis for the new medical curriculum. In Göttingen, for example, future physicians were required to perform "anatomical demonstrations to display their facility for carrying out dissections" before receiving their degree; a skill set that formerly was the exclusive domain of the surgeons.[16] Four of Boerhaave's students, Drs. Andrew St. Clair, John Rutherford, Andrew Plummer, and John Innes, founded the new medical school in Edinburgh in 1726, becoming its first professors in practical medicine and chemistry.[17] Following its establishment, Edinburgh's faculty trained the men who became the tsar's personal physicians into the nineteenth century. From that position, those men planned Russia's curriculum for its surgeons and apothecaries and influenced its hiring practices for those physicians who worked in the Academy of Sciences, the Russian army and navy, and in its major cities.

By the middle of eighteenth century, the medical curriculum across much of Europe was standardized following Leiden's example. It began with "anatomy and physiology, along with botany and chemistry; then general and special pathology, two subjects that taught the causes and classification of disease in general and particular, along with student of *materia medica* and their actions on the body." This would be followed by hands-on experience, in "general and special therapy, clinical practice, the method for writing prescriptions, and specialized courses in surgery, obstetrics, and forensic medicine."[18] Even the comedic handbook for Edinburgh's medical students, *A Guide for Gentlemen Studying Medicine*, appreciated the diversity of topics. Botany, for example, must be studied so "no medical practitioner will choose to hazard his abilities being called in question by his ignorance of the principles of a science which is vulgarly believed to be necessary, and subservient to the study of medicine."[19] Despite the author's sarcasm, producing knowledgeable physicians may also have led to one of Edinburgh's innovations: By 1750, a course in midwifery was added as part of the practical skills required of its students.[20]

Not all medical schools in the eighteenth century adopted Leiden's curriculum or its broad approach to medical science. In France, in particular, its schools resisted the incorporation of surgery and hospital visitations into the medical curriculum. As late as the 1750s, French physicians could graduate without ever treating a patient, and, in the first half of the century, French surgeons developed their own curriculum to support their continuation as a separate discipline from that of the physicians.[21] Russia's preference for Boerhaavian-influenced curricula over the French model, therefore, provided Russia with physicians who had practical experience. It may not have only been the schools these men were trained in that was significant but also the actual training that was key to their hiring.

Practical skills were not the sole key to this curriculum, as the training in nosology, botany, and chemistry all highlighted the value of taxonomic approaches in the history of medicine. Nosology and its taxonomy were central to the relationship between Carl Linnaeus and Boerhaave. The historian Lisa Rosner suggested that Linnaeus "may well have believed that his nosological system described different species of disease," even if other proponents of nosology were not as convinced.[22] Evidence suggests that even Linnaeus may have believed himself to be Boerhaave's chosen successor.[23] With Boerhaave's implicit influence on Linnaeus, students of the Leiden school had a preference for the Linnaean system rather than the competing system of classification that became popular in France, as posited by Georges-Louis Leclerc, the comte de Buffon. Because of the different medical curricula in the early eighteenth century, each group of physicians promoted different classification systems, with Russia's Leiden-influenced group clearly in the Linnaean camp.

Buffon's system of classification was a viable alternative to the Linnaean system in the eighteenth century, even if the latter came to dominate in the nineteenth century. For many, Buffon's system simply seemed more logical. Buffon argued "that only species were truly natural and that all the other categories Linnaeus used—classes, order, genera—were imaginary constructs."[24] His criticism was quite effective in the eighteenth century, which certainly raised doubts about the effectiveness of Linnaeus's system. Physicians and surgeons trained in France, therefore, may have shared an interest with their colleagues in the Netherlands and Germany in the classification of plants, animals, and peoples, but they applied a different set of principles to these groups. It goes too far to suggest that two separate classification schema were at work in the eighteenth century, as these men were in communication with each other, but different strands of identifying principles were familiar to graduates of these two sets of medical schools.[25] For this reason French physicians and natural scientists frequently relied on other French men to produce their classification tables, and German physicians and naturalists relied on other Germans who worked in the alternate system. The organizing principles were simply different.[26]

The Russian state had a clear preference for students from Leiden and its associated universities and programs. Therefore, French physicians, and Buffon's classification schema, never held great influence among the Russian scientific community. Russia's view of its own empire was grounded in the work of Boerhaave, Linnaeus, and the men influenced by their work. Linnaeus had extensive contacts with botanists working in Russia throughout his career, and some of his students would work for the Russian Academy of Sciences.[27] It should not be a surprise, therefore, to note that few, if any, French physicians were working in Russia in the eighteenth century, even during the second half of the century when the University of Paris produced more physicians than any other institution in Europe. This is not to suggest that the men working for the Russian Empire were less well trained than those trained at a French establishment might have been, but rather to highlight that their educational background predisposed their familiarity for some practices more than others.

Russia's Practitioners

Medical practitioners in Russia were hired from one of two established tracks. From one track, university-educated physicians were generally trained in Europe and hired by the Russian state to practice inside the empire. Although many of the men in this group were foreign, dozens of men born inside the empire traveled to Europe for a medical education. These educated, formally trained practitioners in Russia were well familiar with the latest medical theories and therapies, and remained in regular contact with their colleagues in the West, frequently through their alma mater or its publications. On the other track, surgeons and apothecaries were typically trained and practiced at home in Russia, sometimes by working with Western medical professionals and sometimes not. This path should not be mistaken for a divide between foreign and Russian (or local) medical knowledge. This was one community of practitioners at work. Local medicines and drugs arriving in Russian markets from the countryside were as valuable to medical practitioners as those from abroad, and Russia's foreign medical community was often in search of local remedies for local diseases.[28] The Pharmaceutical Chancellery (*Aptekarskii Prikaz*) had a library of Western medical and scientific texts in the seventeenth century, but this did not mean that other forms of knowledge were neglected.[29] Wealth and access to medical treatment, however, did create a barrier for some. Peasants were unlikely to encounter Western-educated physicians, much less a Russian-trained surgeon, but urban residents of all ranks may have benefited from the diagnostic skill of local apothecaries.

Even at the beginning of the seventeenth century, Russia's tsars relied on Western, typically English, physicians for their personal treatment, but under Tsar Peter I Alekseevich, it expanded to include Dutch physicians. During Peter's first Grand Embassy to Europe, he observed medical procedures in the anatomical theater of Dr. Frederik Ruysch in September 1697 in Amsterdam.[30] After the embassy, Ruysch remained one of Peter's correspondents, and the tsar would also visit him in person in 1716 during his second embassy to Europe in addition to meeting Boerhaave at Leiden. During the second embassy, Peter finalized the arrangements to purchase Ruysch's entire scientific collection, including "animals, dried plants, and human anatomical preparations," which were brought back to St. Petersburg to become part of the collection at the new Kunstkamera, which held Peter's cabinet of curiosities.[31] Ruysch's collection was not the only Dutch scientific-material purchase during the second embassy. Peter also visited the apothecary Albertus Seba, having purchased Seba's collection of animal specimens the year before. Ruysch's bill of sale was signed by Seba and Dr. Laurentius Blumentrost, one of Peter's court physicians, and soon to be the head of the Kunstkamera and president of the College of Medicine.[32] Blumentrost was a former student of Ruysch's, demonstrating the influence of this Amsterdam network on both medicine and natural science in Russia.[33]

Nor was Blumentrost alone. Andrei Matveev, Peter's envoy to Amsterdam, hired Nicolaas Bidloo in 1702; Bidloo was another of Ruysch's former students. Bidloo arrived in Russia in 1703 to serve as Peter's personal physician and would establish the first medical training hospital in Moscow in 1706, complete with an anatomy theater and botanical gardens, which became the central office for training Russian surgeons.[34] In addition to the Ruysch connection, Bidloo was also a correspondent of Boerhaave, perhaps arranging the tsar's visit to Boerhaave and his botanical garden in Leiden in 1716. Some historians have suggested Bidloo's Moscow Hospital School was the first medical education institution established in the country, but surgeons had been trained in Moscow for more than half a century before Bidloo's new school.[35] It is more accurate to say that it was the first institution based on Boerhaave's methods in Russia. Its first instructors, alongside Bidloo, were all Dutch and German physicians, with the support of an apothecary and another botanist. It would take some years before the first hospital school gained influence on Russian medical practice. Although the school was built to house and train fifty students, it did not reach that number for more than a decade after it opened its doors.[36]

The Dutch influence was strong, but the Russian government did not exclude other innovative practitioners in Peter's reign. Dr. Robert Areskine was a Scottish physician, who studied under the apothecary Hugh Paterson in Edinburgh for six years, and then completed his MD at University of Utrecht.[37] Areskine became a fellow of the Royal Society of London in 1703 and entered Russian service the following year. Within a few months of arriving in Russia, he was appointed both the head of Pharmaceutical Chancellery and as Peter the Great's personal physician. Before his death in 1718, he had also established the first library in the Kunstkamera in St. Petersburg. From his position of authority, he sponsored other Scots for positions in the Russian government.[38] After his first cousin, John Areskine, the earl of Mar, joined the Jacobite rebellion against King George I in 1714, there were calls on Dr. Areskine to protect other rebels with new occupations in Russia. Several of these men, logically, were physicians, and others served as surgeons for the army during the Great Northern War (1700–1721).[39] Dr. Areskine died at a young age in 1718, and much of his estate remained in Russia to support its new medical foundations. He bequeathed his disposable cash to the Moscow Hospital School to support Bidloo's enterprise, and his personal medical library was added to the collection in the Kunstkamera.[40] Both bequests contributed to the growing Dutch-Scottish influence on the medical establishment.

The Moscow Hospital School trained the majority of medical practitioners working in Russia, alongside the later foundations of the St. Petersburg and Kronstadt schools. These schools did not produce doctors of medicine, but rather *podlekary* (healers or medics-in-training). After a set term of service in the army, these practitioners would receive the title, and increased pay, of a *lekar* (medic). The curriculum in place at each school was the initial one designed by Bidloo for Moscow.[41] Despite the significant numbers of Russian-educated surgeons, it would not be until the 1790s that the Moscow Hospital School would award its first MD. Therefore, even while most of the practicing surgeons in the empire in the eighteenth century were trained in Russia, the MDs at work in the empire were foreign educated. These Russian surgeons were trained in the latest Western techniques, but their position was subservient to those men trained outside the empire who held the rank of physician. Although the Leiden curriculum eroded the traditional divide between educated physician and trained surgeon in its practices, the Russian medical system maintained a version of this divide for most of the eighteenth century.

Any examination of the medical practitioners in Russia in the eighteenth century can hardly fail to note the empire's significant reliance on physicians educated abroad, most of whom were foreign but some were subjects of the empire who sought the medical training available in the West.[42] Competing indexes offer different total numbers of the men at work in Russia during that period. I rely on historian A. B. Bogdanov, whose dataset included the fewest physicians of the various reconstructions, making his numbers the minimum size of the overall community.[43] Bogdanov identified 626 men working in the country during the century; of these, 387 (61.8%) were physicians (MDs), and 165 (26.3%) were surgeons or medics (*chirug*, *lekar*, or *shtab-lekar*). The remaining seventy-eight (12.5%) were part of the medical community but held a variety of posts; some were personal physicians (*leib-medik*), some were generically designated as doctors (*vrach*) but did not hold an MD, and others were assorted members of Russia's Academy of Sciences. This latter group included botanists and chemists who investigated drugs or translated works from abroad. Bogdanov's survey relied on state records as evidence, which did not account for all personal physicians for members of the elite, foreigners acting as merchants inside Russia with medical training, or any type of local healer who may have been in practice. Furthermore, even the recorded men may be considered to provide a low estimate of the total numbers of practitioners, because of the difficulty in documenting when these men entered service or were in practice. The Napoleonic Wars at the turn of the nineteenth century, for example, saw the sudden arrival of numerous new surgeons working for the Russian navy and army; it is likely, however, that some of these men had practiced medicine before 1800. More notably, Bogdanov identified more physicians than surgeons at work in Russia. If these numbers were fully accurate, and not a low estimate, Russia's medical community would be unlike those active in Europe, where, for example, "according to one estimate, for every university graduate in medicine in late-eighteenth-century Germany, twelve practical surgeons were in practice, along with an undetermined number of other healers."[44]

Even with these the caveats, 387 MDs working in Russia in the eighteenth century is a substantial group of trained experts at work inside the empire. At the beginning of the eighteenth century, only a handful of institutions in Europe could bestow an MD. Even some prominent institutions that would play a key role in the eighteenth century did not award degrees for several decades. The University of Edinburgh, for example, which trained most of the tsars' personal physicians during the century, did not grant an MD until 1726.[45] In addition, many of the institutions that could graduate a confirmed MD awarded the degree to only a few men each year. Only a small number of schools graduated more than ten MDs per year at any point in the eighteenth century.[46] Therefore, even with Bogdanov's data providing a low estimate of Russia hiring approximately three new MDs per year for the century, even three physicians per year equated to the government hiring the entire graduating class of some of the smaller medical schools. Although historians have suggested Russia's medical establishment may not have been large, its membership is roughly concurrent with most states in Europe of that era.[47]

The institutions that produced Russia's MDs make a broad list of most medical schools in Europe in the eighteenth century. Of the 387 men Bogdanov identified with an MD, all but 14 include the institutions granting their degree (see table 2.1).

In addition, the universities training these physicians did not steadily supply men to Russia across the century. In general, the institutions

Table 2.1. Degree-granting institutions for Russia's physicians

NUMBER OF PHYSICIANS IN RUSSIA	DEGREE-GRANTING INSTITUTIONS
74	Göttingen
66	Leiden
49	Jena
46	Halle
35	Strasbourg
24	Konigsberg
10	Erfurt
8 from each	Edinburgh and Erlangen
7	Moscow
6 from each	Leipzig and Tubingen
4 from each	Padua and Uppsala
3 from each	Kiel and London
2 from each	Rostock and Utrecht
1 from each	Florence, Greifswald, Hamburg, Krakow, Mecklenburg, and Vilnius

Table 2.2. Russia's physicians hired by decade

DECADE	NUMBER OF PHYSICIANS HIRED
1700–1709	7
1710–1719	6
1720–1729	3
1730–1739	10
1740–1749	18
1750–1759	36
1760–1769	35
1770–1779	40
1780–1789	77
1790–1799	131

with the highest number of graduates at work in Russia (Göttingen, Leiden, Jena, and Halle) sent men consistently throughout the century. Moscow did not bestow this degree until 1791, so its seven MDs in the eighteenth century were not hired until the 1790s (table 2.2).

The notable absence from even a single physician hired from Paris is evidence of how thoroughly the Russian government avoided French-trained physicians. Leiden, under Boerhaave's direction at the beginning of the eighteenth century, was more important than Paris, but its status declined over the course of the century. It is clear from these institutions that Russia's preference was for men trained by Leiden, the schools associated with its curriculum (Göttingen, Jena, Halle, and Edinburgh among them), and generally for institutions in the German-speaking parts of Europe over those elsewhere. Scholars of the eighteenth century have suggested a close connection between France and Russia because of the commonality of speaking French for Russian elites, but Russia's medical establishment had far more in common with Prussia's College of Medicine, which drew extensively on physicians from Halle and Jena, than it did with any French institution.[48]

French members of the Russian Academy of Sciences as well as French natural scientists accompanied one or more of the academy's expeditions during the century, but French physicians did not play a significant role in the medical community in Russia.[49] There are several possibilities why French physicians were unpopular in Russia, but perhaps the most convincing is France's distant relationship with Russia throughout the century. Russia's prominent trade partners in Europe (Britain, the Netherlands, and northern Germany) featured quite prominently, which at least suggests that the towns in which Russia had an established connection were far more likely to send men to Russia.[50] Another consideration may be the French rejection of broadly training its physicians, as surgeons were trained separately. The French reliance on Buffon's classification system may have been equally problematic if most of the medical community would have been trained in the Boerhaave-Linnaean tradition.

The Russian government did send its own subjects abroad to receive specialized training, including medicine. Sixteen men were sent to Leiden for medical training in the 1760s (the peak decade in the century), and twelve would receive their degrees. All of them returned to take positions in the administration, but not only as doctors. Those who did take medical positions became the first Russian-born men to become professors of medicine in Russia, according to historian Nicholas Hans.[51] Petr Dmitrievich Veniaminov was born in Moscow in 1733, began his education in Moscow, but received his MD from Leiden in 1764, completing a thesis on "Uncovering Medical Homicide." Upon his return to Russia, he became a professor at Moscow University. Semen Gerasimovich Zybelin was born in 1735 in Russia and began his education as a student at the Moscow Spiritual Academy.[52] He later studied medicine at Konigsberg, Berlin, and eventually received his MD at Leiden in 1764 with a thesis on "Medicinal Substances, and Their Natural Diversity and Chemical Principles for Medical Use." He became a professor of medicine at Moscow University in 1765. These Leiden students were not the only Russians trained abroad in this period. Aleksei Protas'evich Protasov, for example, was born in St. Petersburg in 1725, studied in a seminary in Russian in the 1740s, and joined the Academy of Sciences in 1750. Following that appointment, he went abroad to study medicine at Strasbourg, completing his MD in 1763 with a thesis on "Anatomic-Physiological Basis for the Action of Ingested Substances in the Human Stomach."

The likelihood of Russian subjects who studied medicine abroad to return to the empire was quite high, but they were not the only men at work in Russia in the eighteenth century. Working abroad in the eighteenth century was an unusual choice. Physicians frequently worked near to their academic institutions, as it was easiest to study and work in an environment in which they would be familiar "with the local customs, religion, and dialect," as well as cultivate useful contacts.[53] For the Russian subjects who studied abroad, returning home to an appointment eased this transition. It is more difficult to explain, however, those men born in the West who opted for careers in Russia. Studying in Jena, for example, and working in St. Petersburg, could be lucrative but would make returning home to Jena only more difficult. Many of the physicians who worked in Russia relied on their personal networks and connections for their positions.

Johann Amman reflected how successfully these networks could operate. Amman was born in Switzerland and received an MD from Leiden, before beginning his professional career in 1730 as the curator of Dr. Hans Sloane's botanical collection in London.[54] Sloane was a member of both Royal College of Physicians and the Royal Society, serving as president of both for lengthy terms. Aside from his positions, he was a well-known naturalist, with a correspondence network that spanned Europe and crossed the Atlantic.[55] Amman became a fellow of the Royal Society in 1731, and then entered Russian service as the curator for the Kunstkamera's botanical collection in 1733. Although Amman died young at age thirty-four, during his eight years in Russia, he forged a personal union between the Royal Society and the Russian Academy. Amman sent Sloane samples of minerals, seeds, and dried plants, as well as descriptions and illustrations of animals, to add materials from the Volga Region, the Caucasus, and Siberia to Sloane's collection, which famously became the core collection at the British Museum. Sloane also acted as a hub of connections, as he corresponded with naturalists and physicians across Europe. In his files, letters from Amman sit next to letters from Linnaeus and Boerhaave.[56]

The Amman-Sloane connection proved pivotal in maintaining the relationship between the Royal Society in London and the Russian Academy of Sciences. Sloane regularly sent two copies of each new volume of the Society's *Philosophical Transactions* to Amman. Amman kept one for his personal library, and the second was presented to the academy's president for its library. Frequently, the texts were accompanied by seeds, sometimes those specifically requested by Amman and at other times seeds that Sloane thought would be of interest or potentially useful. For example, in a letter from March 1736, Amman thanked Sloane for the *Transactions*, as well as copies of a "Chinese Chronology" that would be donated to the library, and he requested seeds of two types of South American balsam trees, copaiba and tolu, and "true Ipecacuanha," for his garden in St. Petersburg.[57] Amman also requested specific titles that were desired by various members of the Academy of Sciences, including Mark Catesby's *Natural History of California, Florida, and Bahama Islands*, *The Whole Works of Walter Moyle, Esq.*; William Petty's

"A Treatise on Taxes & Contributions, shewing the Nature and Measures of Crown Lands, . . ."; and Dr. Martin Lister's *Historiae sive synopsis methodica conchyliorum*, a study of shells from the Caribbean.[58] Sloane made a successful book agent, arranging for the texts to be purchased in London and then delivered to St. Petersburg by members of the Russia Company, most often William Vigor, who regularly appears in the correspondence as a trusted friend of both men.[59]

Although Amman trusted his former mentor, Sloane, as a reliable source of information, Amman did not blindly accept all the information the network provided. In particular, Amman remained skeptical of Linnaeus's new taxonomy system, objecting to Linnaeus's choice to sex plants, as other botantists did.[60] He wrote: "I have received lately from Dr. Gronovius at Leden some Systematical tables concerning natural History, composed by Dr. Linnaeus. His botanical tables are in my opinion more curious than useful & I doubt very much if any Botanist will follow his lewd method. Why does he not take his Systematical disposition of Animals from their Cuanus & Penis as well as in the plants, since those parts have the very some use in fructification, which is according to the Doctor's observations on the Regnum vegetabile, the chief vue the Creator had in producing them."[61] The criticism may be consistent with the views of Linnaeus's earliest iterations of the taxonomic system, and this reaction is why Linnaeus continued to produce revisions for a few decades. Although later members of the academy would be more receptive to the system, Linnaeus's first draft was not well received.[62]

Amman's major scientific contribution while in St. Petersburg was his monograph on plants native to the "Tatarian, Siberian, & Davurian" parts of the Russian Empire. This work was illustrated with plates produced by the academy's engraver.[63] Although "several descriptions [were] made only from dry specimens," Amman continued to make revisions while waiting for publication to be printed. In 1738, he had "received lately a pretty large parcel of Seeds, gathered near Samara on the river Wolga, & Olecminskoi & Kirensko Ostroy on the river Len, between Iakutsh & Irtusk" that he hoped to include, even if he did "not know as yet for the most part, what they are."[64] Amman grew all of these specimens in his personal garden in St. Petersburg, as the academy was resistant to establishing one of its own. He remarked more than once that this was unlike the College of Medicine, which was currently enjoyed a revival of its gardens, not only in St. Petersburg but also in Moscow and Astrakhan.[65]

There was widespread interest across Europe in Amman's botanical work, including from Linnaeus. Once Amman reached St. Petersburg, he and Linnaeus were in regular correspondence, sharing materials and texts on botany. Considering Amman's reaction to the first edition of *Systema Naturae*, it was occasionally uneasy, particularly in comparison to the far more cordiale letters Amman sent to his former mentor in London. When Amman wrote to Linnaeus the month after receiving the text, he acknowledged his receipt of it, but failed to mention his thoughts on its inappropriateness, despite sharing them a month earlier with Sloane.[66] The following year, a common associate in the Netherlands shared Amman's objections to sexing plants, leading Amman to apologize to Linnaeus for sharing his criticism of the taxonomy with the botanical community without informing Linnaeus directly of his concerns.[67]

While Amman was among Russia's best-connected naturalists, he was not alone in sharing the ongoing scientific work across Europe. John Bell, a Scottish physician who entered Russian service in 1714, had a decades-long career in Russia, acting for the Russian and British governments at times. He was recommended for service by Peter the Great's personal physician, Robert Areskine. Shortly after arriving in Russia, Bell was dispatched on Artemii Petrovich Volynskii's embassy to Iran in 1716. Volynskii's mission was to negotiate a new trade agreement, but Bell's was to investigate medical practices in the Middle East.[68] Bell's success, unlike Volynskii's, resulted in him joining an embassy sent to China in 1719 under the direction of Lev Vasilevich Izmailov. By the 1730s, Bell was operating as a trusted member of the Russia Company in St. Petersburg, on occasion advising the British consul on economic matters.[69] Bell published a lengthy narrative of his travels to China and Iran upon his return to Scotland in the 1760s, including a discussion of medical practices in Iran and China as well as Russia's commercial interests in each region.[70] In his final years in Scotland, Bell acted as an intermediary in the botanical exchanges between Dr. John Hope, the head of the Royal Botanic Garden of Edinburgh and fellow of the Royal Academy, and Dr. Peter Simon Pallas in Russia.[71]

Pallas was born in Berlin and was educated at Halle and Göttingen before receiving his medical degree from Leiden in 1760. In 1767, he became a member of the Russian Academy of Sciences and led a scientific expedition into Siberia to record new plants across the empire. Upon his return to St. Petersburg, he became Russia's leading botanist. It is no wonder that he was a desirable correspondent for John Hope, and Bell's intervention established a personal connection between these men. Nor was the Hope-Bell-Pallas connection isolated, as studying with Hope at University of Edinburgh became one path toward employment in Russia. This was the case for both Dr. Danila Iakovlevich Pischekov, who was born in Sloboda, Ukraine, and graduated from Edinburgh in 1784, and Dr. Iurii Aleksandrovich Bakhmet'ev, who was born in Moscow and graduated from Edinburgh in 1786.

Russian recruitment of its physicians from Europe fell into predictable channels of preferring the graduates from a few selected schools, which emphasized certain medical traditions over others. The legacy of Boerhaave's curriculum, which underlay the curricula at Edinburgh and Göttingen, was an integrated study of medical theory and practical experience in botany, surgery, and treating patients in hospitals. It is not a surprise that the Russian government revised its medical curriculum for its hospital training schools to follow this example. Doing so reinforced Russia's preference to recruit those men produced by the schools that shared a similar curriculum to their preferred institutions.

Professional Networks

During Peter the Great's reign, personal networks successfully brought trained professionals to Russia. Robert Areskine hired John Bell; Areskine and Bell were both trained in Edinburgh before receiving their MDs on the Continent. Another example would be Dr. Daniel Gottlieb Messerschmidt who studied botany and medicine in Jena and Halle, the latter from which he received his doctorate in 1713. One of Messerschmidt's instructors at Halle was also a fellow of the Royal Academy in London, who introduced him to Robert Areskine, who in turn hired Messerschmidt to work at the Kunstkamera in 1718. Shortly thereafter, Peter the Great personally assigned Messerschmidt to investigate Siberian plants under the direction of Dr. Laurentius Blumentrost, Ruysch's former student.[72] Samples that Messerschmidt sent to St. Petersburg from Siberia were occasionally dispatched to London by Amman, where Siberian plants still remain in the Sloane herbarium.[73] Messerschmidt, in other words, was perfectly positioned to prosper in Russia, with an immediate connection to both professional pools from which Peter's government hired. He also demonstrated the value of the universities in Jena and Halle, which came to dominate the ranks of Russia's physicians over the course of the century.

Shortly after Messerschmidt's arrival, new laws addressed the improvement of Russia's medical practice, with the outcome of reorganizing the older Pharmaceutical Chancellery to become the new College of Medicine, which supervised not only the old office but also the Moscow Hospital School.[74] In April 1721, as part of a broad bill affecting all of the Swedes in Russian service, the state required surgical and apothecary manuals to be translated into Russian to make the material readily accessible. In addition, practitioners were required to have the approval of the recently appointed head of the Kuntskamera and president of the College of Medicine, Blumentrost.[75] In August 1721, the Senate extended the college's reach to include supervising the purchase of all *materia medica* down to the district level, providing the new college the right to intervene in all medical practice in the country.[76] It was not clear if the new college would have had sufficient staff for this level of oversight, but in theory, Blumentrost's office was expected to confirm the quality of all medicaments available in Russia. Neither law comprehensively addressed the requirements for training staff nor set a curriculum of set topics. In fact, it recognized that Russia's surgeons and apothecaries were trained in country, whereas the supervising physicians were educated abroad. This educational background not only would divide the physicians from the other practitioners but also expected the surgeons and apothecaries to be trained in Russian, which was not required for physicians. Blumentrost's new position, including his extensive supervisory role, raised Messerschmidt's profile alongside his own.[77]

Messerschmidt's career in Russia demonstrates how personal connections served state interests by promoting Russia as a center for research and its potential contributions to the work of early-modern naturalists and physicians. Messerschmidt was recommended to Areskine for Russian employment by Dr. Johann Philipp Breyne, who was fellow of the Royal Society and the German Academy of Sciences Leopoldina. Breyne had been proposed for Royal Society membership by Sloane in 1703. When Peter the Great's government dispatched Messerschmidt to Siberia to investigate its natural resources, the government took advantage of his findings and also established a route for promoting Russia's scientific work across Europe.

On Messerschmidt's expedition, he would travel as far east as Lake Baikal, gathering plants and minerals for further investigation. As a new arrival to Russia, much less its far eastern empire, Messerschmidt relied on a local network of experts to inform his investigation.[78] Although it is certain that both Russians and Siberians assisted the official scientific expedition, Messerschmidt also relied on information provided by a Swedish prisoner of war, Philip Johan von Strahlenberg, who lived in exile in Tobol'sk from 1711 to 1721. According to Strahlenberg's biographer, while in Siberia, Strahlenberg was in correspondence with Breyne in Germany, who likely provided an introduction for Messerschmidt.[79] Strahlenberg would later publish his own account of Siberia's resources upon his return to Sweden, but when these two men crossed paths in 1721 in Tobol'sk, their exchange of knowledge influenced Messerschmidt's investigation.[80] Messerschmidt died at a young age before he officially published any of his fieldwork, but his research still appeared in print, through the intercession of Breyne and Sloane.[81]

While Messerschmidt was still in Siberia on his expedition, Sloane published an article in the Royal Society's *Philosophical Transactions* on a hotly contested topic for naturalists—that is, whether mammoth bones were the remains of ancient animals or a new type of naturally occurring mineral. In his "Account of the elephants teeth and bones found under ground" in 1728, Sloane began with a discussion of the tusk he had received from Bell and mentioned how "other Bones of the same Animal, that is, of the Elephant, are found in sundry Parts of Siberia to a considerable Quantity, and the Tusks and Teeth in particular, when less corrupted, are used all over Russia for Ivory." In his article, Sloane offered no definite conclusion on the origin of the bones but had hopes that further research would prove that "these Bones are the Bones, and the Horns, . . . of Elephants drowned in the universal Deluge."[82]

Messerschmidt's fieldwork provided a potential answer for Sloane's inquiry. In 1738, Breyne published portions of Messerschmidt's notes and illustrations in *Philosophical Transactions* with Sloane's support. Breyne's conclusion was that Messerschmidt's research proved mammoths were elephants, agreeing with Sloane.[83] The agreement did not come as a surprise; after all, the connection between Breyne and Sloane was the reason Areskine hired Messerschmidt. These men were clearly in close contact. Equally important, Messerschmidt may not have lived long enough to see the results of his research published in Europe's leading journals, but this personal network fulfilled that project for him. Historians of science viewed this connection leading to publication as the operation of a "trust network" of correspondents.[84] Information was easier to accept if the original source was known as reliable; personal connections were best, but letters of introduction from trusted informants or contracts could forge new bonds. Information arriving from less familiar contacts were more suspect. Messerschmidt's advisor, Breyne, shared the informed the man who recommended him for membership in the Royal Society, Sloane. Messerschmidt did not have an opportunity to prepare the material for publication, but, having sent letters and notes to Breyne, the Royal Society published this material in *Philosophical Transactions*. The Royal Society regularly sent its publication to all of the scientific academies in Europe, sending Messerschmidt's observations on a remarkable journey—from Siberia to Breyne in Germany to Sloane in London to St. Petersburg's Academy.

Although Sloane and Breyne clearly valued Messerschmidt's contributions, not all members of the academy were as pleased with his fieldwork. Sloane requested Amman provide copies of Messerschmidt's notes so the material could be published in *Philosophical Transactions*, but Amman declined in 1739. Amman wrote: "I think it will not be worth while to have them [the notes] copied for you; since I have begun to draw out of them the most remarquables observations in order to publish them by degrees. This man is so prolix & tedious in his descriptions of birds & four footed animals, that there is a hardly any pin or hair, wch he hath not measured."[85] Amman's death interrupted his plans to exploit Messerschmidt's information, but his objections demonstrated that sharing information was not a simple process.

Despite Amman's objections, the publication of a portion of Messerschmidt's notes was important for the Russian government. As the state increased its investment in both hiring foreign specialists and investigating its natural resources (albeit people, animals, plants, or minerals), this type of publication and its very public reception had value for Russia's reputation. The progress of Messerschmidt's work from Siberia to publication in London demonstrated the growing interest in Russia as a naturalists' laboratory. For individuals pursuing careers in Russia, the process by which Messerschmidt, a German doctor, was hired and utilized by Russia, demonstrated how a career in Russia could advance an international reputation, even if Messerschmidt passed away before his work appeared in print. It should not be a surprise that during the 1720s, Russia established its own Academy of Sciences, as well as its own publication, *Commentarii Academiae Scientiarum Imperialis Petropolitanae*. This was a logical step in supporting the establishment of Russia's scientific reputation, mirroring the apparatus established elsewhere, including in London.

By the 1730s, Russia's College of Medicine formalized the medical establishment; the Kunstkamera and the Academy of Sciences regulated the naturalists' investigations. Each of these acts undertaken by the

Russian government represented a significant investment of resources in an era in which the state scrambled for new economic opportunities. Peter the Great's reign with its substantial outlays for his decades of war and establishment of the new capital, among other projects, was a major setback for Russia's finances. Therefore, investing in science and medicine was not done solely in pursuit of demonstrating Russia's ability to lead scientific inquiries; it was increasingly apparent that damage to Russia's reputation was possible if Russia's experts did not lead these conversation. John Bernard Müller, a Swedish captain taken as a prisoner of war, lived in Tobol'sk in 1716. He later produced a memoir of his time in the Russian Empire focused on the populations of Siberia, who remained relatively unknown to Western scholars. He was intrigued by the prevalence of scurvy among the Ostiaks, who suffered from a general bodily rot "not much unlike a Leprosy." Furthermore, he noted that the Ostiaks lacked "Self-preservation . . . to such a degree, that when any such Distemper appears either upon a Foot, the Back, or any other part of the Body, even the Face, they do not apply any other Remedy, but suffer the Corruption to spread till their very Bones are rotten, and the Disease ends with their Lives." Muller believed the Ostiaks' scurvy was the result of their lack of hygiene, poor diet, and general immorality, as seen in their "irregular Desires," which led to "nothing but Licentiousness and Confusion."[86] In the Russian Empire, immoral habits threatened the physical well-being of imperial subjects. The future of the empire depended on improving not only health but also customs and lifestyles.

Müller was not alone. Strahlenberg, the Swedish prisoner of war who acted as one of Messerschmidt's Siberian consultants, published an assessment of Siberia's people and resources in 1730, shortly after the establishment of the new Academy of Sciences. It was hardly unusual for visitors to Russia to publish an account of their experiences, or for those like Jodocus Crull, who had never been to Russia, to summarize others' views. Strahlenberg's account, however, arrived after he served as a local consultant for a Russian-hired physician working as part of a state-planned scientific expedition. Russia, accidently perhaps, made Strahlenberg an expert, but one who most definitely was not on the state's payroll.

Strahlenberg's narrative aspired to provide a comprehensive view of the Russia's history, government, society, and geography, climate, and resources.[87] He had been a long-term resident in Siberia because of his exile, unlike men like Samuel Collins who had been a resident but never traveled beyond the Urals. Strahlenberg was clear from the beginning that he disagreed with earlier Russian descriptions. "Of the Climate of *Russia* several Accounts have been given in Books of Geography and Travels, But as the Ancients depended pretty much, on the Intelligence that got of Foreigners, and mostly from Hearsay only; And our more modern Writers, in this Point, as in many others, have blindly followed them, without any farther due Examination." If the consensus from the seventeenth century was that Russia's extreme cold was its dominant feature, Strahlenberg dissented: "When they say, in general: *Russia* is very cold, and lies in a raw Climat, has longer Winters than Summers, and is, on Account of the vast Forests it contains, very little cultivated; Such general Accounts must not be look'd upon, as applicable to the whole Country." Instead, Strahlenberg viewed Russia as having four climatological zones, from the northern taiga that was dominated by its cold winters to the southern steppe: "Countries have a very warm and temperate Air, and short Winters. The whole Extent of this Country is flat and even, has little Morass, is water'd by many Rivers, and abounds in Fish."[88] Certainly, Strahlenberg's assessment of the empire as temperate broke with the earlier narratives' depiction of Russia's extreme conditions.

Strahlenberg's positive description of the climate and conditions of the steppe became the first of several implicit, and at times explicit, critiques of Russia's management of its lands. In a section on Siberia, for example, Russia's failure was obvious: "As to the Rivers in *Siberia*, they have naturally a pretty good Communication with one another; So that it is easy to come from one into the other. However, there are two Places, which might with a little Labour be cut thro', by which a great Circuit would be avoided in going to *China*, as well as to *Mungolia*; But few People living on those Spots, and not many coming thither, they have not been observed; And besides, Colonies must first be establish'd there, before such a Work could be undertaken."[89] Siberia could be productive, "with a little Labour," but Russia's failure to colonize the region left it wild and untamed, waiting for someone to exploit its potential.

And its potential was vast, as Strahlenberg documented in extraordinary detail in his remarkable chapter, "Of the most noted Mercantile and Fair-Towns, as also of the Mines, Minerals, Vegetables, Fossils, Curiosities, Antiquities, Manufactures, Fabricks, &c. in the Russian Empire, digested into Alphabetical Order." In about one hundred pages, Strahlenberg summarized not only the animal, plant, and mineral resources of Siberia but also its Indigenous peoples, who were another resource waiting to be properly exploited by a more capable government. In this, he predicted much of the criticism waiting for the Russian Empire in the eighteenth century, especially from French physiocrats who highlighted Russia's inability to control its most valuable resource, its subjects.[90] Russia's failure with its non-Russian peoples were persistent, not the least of which because most remained "heathen Nation[s]," in Strahlenberg's parlance. One of those "heathens," the Baraba Tatars, lived "between the Cities of *Tara* and *Tomskoi*" and were noted for their "Schamans." The Russians failed to note the most basic facts about these Tatars, according to Strahlenberg: "Formerly they were one and the same Nation with the *Ostiacks*, on the River *Oby*, which both they and the *Barabintzi* told me, when I travell'd through their Country; The District where they live, the Russians, according to their bad Pronunciation of the *Tartarian* Words, call *Barabu*; But the *Tartars* and *Ostiacks* call it *Barama*."[91]

The Iakuts were no more favorably depicted. "*Jakuhti*, Are a *Pagan* People, called so by the *Russians*; They are under the *Russian* Government, and live along the River *Lena*. . . . They have, besides, many superstitious Customs, in common with other Nations, which they celebrate about certain Trees, that they look upon to be sacred." Not only did the Russians once again fail to correctly note the name of this group, who were "their own Tongue, *Zinzacha*, or *Zinzogotock*" but also Russia's experts made errors in describing them. "What *Isbrand Ides* (in his Travels, p. 132) relates, concerning these People, is all true; Excepting the Custom of burying alive, or killing the oldest Servants, or Favourites of a Prince, at his Funeral, which is abolish'd." To prove his point, Strahlenberg detailed the history of the ritual execution and when it had been abandoned, well before Ides's travels in the 1690s. Even if the Iakuts had modified their "pagan" practices, there was little to commend about them. After critiquing their religious practices, society, and lifestyle, Strahlenberg assessed the humoralist necessities: characteristics and food. He wrote: "These people are very nasty; They seldom, or hardly ever, wash themselves; They will eat the Flesh of Oxen, Cows, and Horses, but no Pork, be they never so hungry; But then they never mind whether the Cattle be sick or sound; For they indifferently kill and eat it. . . . They eat Bread, when they can get it, but it is no usual Part of their Diet, because they neither Plough, Sow, nor Plant."[92]

Strahlenberg's detailed description of Siberia critiqued the Russian Empire's lack of influence over the Siberian population. Strahlenberg was no less critical of others who presented themselves as experts on

Siberia. In particular, he rejected Sloane's analysis of mammoth bones, published in *Philosophical Transactions*, based on his communication with one of Russia's physicians, Bell. Strahlenberg's entry on mammoth bones argued he was the only possible expert on the topic: "I have taken a good deal of Pains, during my Travels, to come at some Certainty, with Respect to this Mineral, if I may call it so." Suggesting that the mammoth bones could in fact be a mineral, raised the idea that these were not ancient remains, as Sloane theorized. Explicitly mentioning his connection to Messerschmidt, who observed whole skeletons, Strahlenberg allowed himself to be convinced these were animals, but they were not elephants from before the Biblical Flood as Sloane had argued. Instead, "these Teeth and Bones are of Sea-Animals, such as the Danes formerly us'd to bring from Greenland, and Iceland, and sell for those of Unicorns."[93] When Breyne published Messerschmidt's notes in *Philosophical Transactions* in 1738, it was both a response to Strahlenberg's critique of Sloane and an attempt to validate Messerschmidt's authority.

The success of Strahlenberg's text, reprinted in multiple languages within a decade, demonstrated the demand across Europe for more information about Russia's Empire. A similar text, reputedly by another Swedish prisoner of war, would be published during this era. It appeared in *Tatarie dressee sur les memoires originaux de Suedois prisonniers en Siberie* (1737), and was edited and compiled by its Dutch publisher, Jan Frederic Bernard. The text was translated into English for a British edition by William Farrington the following year, although his translation remained unpublished.[94] Bernard published a series of travel narratives in the far north from 1715 to 1738, making this supposed Swedish account one of the final entries.[95] It is not clear whether Bernard was only the editor of the narrative based on unpublished Swedish narratives, or, if the entire narrative was a fiction. Following Strahlenberg's narrative, however, a "Swedish prisoner" in Russia had the appearance of a reliable source.

Bernard's volume offered a distinct perspective on the Russian Empire or, more specifically, "Grand Tatary," the Eurasian expanse from the Volga River to the Pacific Coast. He offered an exceptional take on the region's geography, suggesting "this vast Country is under the finest Climate of the Universe, & of extraordinary goodness & Fertility, but as it is also one of the higher of the habitable World, it wants Water in Several Places." Elevation and the arid quality of the land was a previously unknown version of Russia's Asia. Furthermore, this geography caused raised specific problems. The first was its climate:

"This great Elevation is the cause that this Country seems very cold in comparison of others under the same Latitude, People of good credit have assured me on the spot that the north wind is there so penetraint even in the midst of summer that they must cover themselves well in the night not to catch Cold." The second was more troubling: Russia's inability to support a sizeable population. Or as Bernard noted: "This great Elevation of Tartary is also the cause that notwithstanding all thos great Rivers which have their Rise there they want Water in several places, so that it cant be inhabited but in the neighbourhood of the Rivers & Lakes. Tis for this Reason also that there are so many desarts, but these desarts to which the Russes give the name of Stepp."[96]

In light of Russia's problematic geography and climate, Bernard assessed its populace as accordingly weakened. He wrote of the Tatars (all of the population between the Volga and the Pacific): "In general they love drink & if they are not perfect drunkards, its rather for Want of Opportunity, than for the Will, for as soon as they can get strong Liquors they never leave off drinking till they fall all along." He was aware that many of Russia's subjects were Muslim, and therefore "by the duty of their Religion to take more care of themselves than the others, & tis for this, they say, that this Fault has been less observed" in the Uzbeks, Circassians, Crimean Tatars, and Baraba Tatars. Bernard noted, however, that this duty of care may not have been from strict adherence to religious precepts as much as "this proceeds more from the Climate which they first live in which is milder & more southerly; We see that the Northern People are naturally inclined to Strong Liquors, & that more or less according as they approach the North."[97] It would be hard to suggest that Bernard did not have a fully developed sense of climate determinism, as in his survey, the climate above all else determined lifestyle. The remaining chapters of his study considered other groups still outside the Russian Empire, including the Bukharans and Mongols, and finished with an analysis of the Turkic languages being spoken across Eurasia. Unlike his antecedents, for Bernard, elevation became the persistent threat to the success of Russia's subjects.

Strahlenberg and Bernard demonstrated the potential danger of allowing narratives of the Russian Empire to be left in the hand of outsiders, including the men who had lived in the empire, but were not on its payroll, as well as the men who had never lived in Russia and possessed, at best, secondhand knowledge of its distinct features and peoples. The insiders, those employees of the state or the tsar, were crafting official narratives and describing its climate, geography, peoples, languages, and lifestyles, as well as its resources, such as animal, mineral, or plant, whereas the outsiders frustrated the official narrative with their own. This is not to suggest that everyone who worked for the Russian Empire was never critical of it or of the state's management of its resources. Amman regularly shared updates on current climatic conditions with Sloane, partially from his astonishment that Russia's extreme cold had not decimated the animal and plant populations. This extreme cold reached its peak in 1739, when it had "been so extraordinary in those regions that . . . I observed with 2 different Thermometers," the temperature was below the level estimated where life could not be sustained. "Nevertheless, animals of all kinds have survived this cold. It is never good to draw consequences of things not yet confirmed by experiments."[98] Amman had raised concerns about the extreme conditions earlier. In 1736, for example, St. Petersburg had suffered from the "most Severe weather . . . wch continued very near 3 weeks; several persons have been found frozen, others lost their Ears or noses." The arrival of the Iranian ambassador with a gift of an elephant for Anna Ivanovna (r. 1730-1740) was delayed by the cold, with the government "oblig'd to make boots for him [the elephant], & [had] to cover him with cloaths, otherwise he had been frozen to death."[99] Like many of his fellow foreigners in St. Petersburg, Amman also believed the climate was ultimately responsible for his declining health. In 1741, shortly before his death, he wrote in his last letter to Sloane, "Concerning my health, of wch you desire to be acquainted, I find it from day to day to decay. I can not bear this extremely rough & inconstant climate."[100]

The large medical community at work in Russia existed within overlapping networks of personal and professional ties. Family members frequently followed fathers or uncles into service. Leading figures in medical education sent several of their students to work in Russia once the network was established. The result of these connections was a communal view of the importance of practical medical education in Russia; a comprehensive system that involved iatrophysical, iatrochemical, nosological, and humoral theories, with the men appropriately practiced in treating patients and employing their knowledge of botany, chemistry, and surgery. Furthermore, and perhaps most important, this was not an isolated community in Russia, but rather one that was fully integrated with the medical institutions that trained these men in the Netherlands, Germany, and Great Britain. Some of these men were the hub of their own personal network, creating connections between Russia and the West. Others were dependent on their personal and professional correspondence to maintain these links, either discussing medical treatment and practice with extended kin networks or by publishing their studies in the leading scientific journals of that era, both in Europe and in Russia, to publicize their contributions to science.

Interest in the role of correspondence in the dissemination of early-modern scientific thought has been a growing area of study for several historians. Lindsay O'Neill has argued that for social historians networks were "webs of social support that undergirded the functioning of local societies," while for historians of science "networks were more fluid, more fragile, and more geographically expansive. They were the product of a shared belief, need, or interest." She has suggested combining the two approaches, because "the deeply entangled nature of the two" has not been explored.[101] This idea had been suggested by other scholars as well. Roy Porter, for example, argued that "the locus of the English medical Enlightenment lay with the private, the individual, the local, the personal, the voluntary," suggesting the need to look beyond professional networks to understand fully the process by which medical was disseminated.[102] Margaret DeLacy agreed, arguing that for some medical issues, it was "the Royal Society that collected information on inoculation, debated it, disseminated information and technical advice, and ultimately initiated a successful campaign to put it into practice," not the London College of Physicians.[103] As Thomas Broman suggested, even when physicians published debates over medical theories and treatments in their professional publications, "the audience for them consisted of that much broader, vaguely defined 'public.' As a consequence, the standard of argument conformed to the universally accessible canons of 'reason,' rather than being accessible only to a privileged clique of specialists."[104]

Therefore, both official and unofficial records exist of the dissemination of medical and climatological knowledge to and from Russia. Official communications include the articles on medicine, botany, and chemistry published in the Russian Academy of Sciences journal, *Commentarii Academiae Scientiarum Imperialis Petropolitanae*, as well as the work of physicians and natural scientists working in Russia that were published in other academies' publication, including the *Philosophical Transactions of the Royal Society of London* and medical school journals.[105] In addition to these scientific journals, many of the men at work in Russia published their research and observations in treatises, ethnographic and botanical studies of the empire, and even travel narratives. The outsiders, those not on the state's payroll, however, published as often about life in the Russian Empire. Perhaps inevitably, those other narratives presented damning assessments of Russia's inability to manage, much less improve, its resources. As a result, intentional or not, when the Academy of Sciences launched its first major scientific expedition, the Second Kamchatka Expedition in 1733, it was investing in an official narrative to counter the criticism from men like Strahlenberg and Bernard.

Caveats aside, a common medical and scientific understanding emerged of the Russian Empire in the eighteenth century. This understanding was based on the curriculum developed at Leiden and supported by Linnaeus's classification system. Selecting men who were trained in this curriculum and the Linnaean system had the endorsement of the Russian government. These foreign hires were not random choices, but rather were men recruited from specific schools. Information created and recorded by this group could be disseminated rapidly through a trust network. Although the Russian Academy of Sciences and College of Medicine were the central hubs of this network in Russia, the material produced by this group would also be published in Russia, Germany, the Netherlands, and Britain. The medical and scientific community of Russia was already fully integrated with Europe, at least for its educated elites.

Part II

Applying Knowledge

CHAPTER 3

Describing Kamchatka, Documenting Scurvy

Travel narratives provided foreigners with an avenue to criticize Russia. If it was not the autocratic government or its reliance on serfdom, it was the meager food or the extreme cold that made it unpalatable. Once men in Russian service began to publish their narratives, descriptions of Russia circulating across Europe's republic of letters became complimentary. The tsars and their government managed a vast empire with extensive resources. The climate may have been extremely cold, but Russians overcame this humoral impediment through their use of the bania, or by their diet, or both. Russian men and women were attractive and procreative, surprising for melancholic or phlegmatic people. The people of the empire, however, were not portrayed as positively. They were frequently depicted as hairless, short, and disinterested in sex, all stereotypically cold features. They lacked the necessary energy or efficiency to manage their resources. This version of the non-Russian people was most often found in Siberia, which remained elusive, beyond the reach of foreign observers.

With the establishment of the Academy of Sciences and the reorganization of the College of Medicine in the 1720s, the Russian government had an opportunity to address this negative view of Siberia and the empire as a whole. When the Swedish prisoners of war, particularly Philipp Johann von Strahlenberg, published critical assessments of Siberia based on their lived experiences in the region, the pressure to respond to their critique increased. The Russian government, and its servitors, were already attempting to redress the lack of knowledge about the region. Laurentius Blumentrost and Daniel Gottlieb Messerschmidt led expeditions to gather materials specifically for this purpose. When the state sponsored the First Kamchatka Expedition in 1725, this was another attempt to document and reveal Russia's success in managing its Asian empire. Once its leader, Vitus Bering, returned to St. Petersburg in 1731 with maps documenting Russia's Pacific coastline, it opened a window on a new region for Russia to exploit. The Second Kamchatka Expedition (1733–1743) was large, involving a staff of hundreds and specialists hired from across Europe. It investigated plants and minerals, peoples and their histories, and documented this process with scientific studies, maps, and physical samples, some of which would be sent to Carl Linnaeus to contribute to his ongoing classification system.

Focusing on the physicians in this chapter, including Johann Georg Gmelin's Siberian observations and his connection to Linnaeus, I add to earlier studies of the Second Kamchatka Expedition's scientific and historical merit by considering the way in which the published narratives reflected the structures of knowledge production, in terms of humoral language and the physicians' professional networks.[1] The expedition relied on humoral descriptions to understand the peoples of Siberia and the North Pacific. This ethnographic information contributed to Linnaeus's taxonomic system, and not only affected the classification schema but also addressed Russia's disease burden.

It should not be a surprise that men from the Russian Academy's favorite institutions, including University of Tübingen, held leadership roles. Nor should it be a surprise that both botanists working for the expedition were not trained as naturalists but rather as physicians, given that Russia preferred professionals who were trained in the Boerhaavian curriculum, which included botany as an essential skill. Disagreements among these men were many, but, by including only those who shared a common educational background, the Russian government encouraged knowledge about the empire into established tracts, including Linnaeus's taxonomy.[2] Even while the Second Kamchatka Expedition made new discoveries about Russia's possessions, this knowledge fit within preexisting parameters.

The Second Kamchatka Expedition

Vitus Jonassen Bering led both the First and Second Kamchatka Expeditions. Born in Denmark, Bering began his naval career at fifteen and joined the Russian navy in 1704. Peter the Great selected him to lead the First Kamchatka Expedition (1725–1731) commissioned to investigate the potential connection between Kamchatka and North America. Bering and his assistants, the Danish Martin Spanberg and the Russian Aleksei Ilyich Chirikov, produced new maps of the coastlines of the North Pacific and proof of the straits that separated Asia from America. Upon his return to St. Petersburg, Bering proposed a more expansive undertaking, which became the Second Kamchatka Expedition (1733–1743).[3]

The first expedition had a crew of fewer than fifty men, whereas the second involved more than three hundred and included a wide array of scientific specialists drawn primarily from the ranks of the Russian Academy. Messerschmidt's fieldwork in Siberia, gathering and identifying new plants and minerals, was ongoing while the First Kamchatka was exploring the North Pacific. For the Second Kamchatka, the naval expedition and scientific mission were combined, but this was not the limit of its ambition. The first instruction to Bering was "to bring the local peoples to the Christian faith."[4] Although no missionary held a prominent role in the expedition, its naturalists documented aspects of religious practice across the empire, focusing on the Muslim and animistic peoples.

In May 1732, a lengthy instruction identified what types of provisions and support should be provided by which towns across Siberia, and explicitly identified peasants from the town of Ilimsk and the nearby Tungus peoples as the target audience to provide manpower.[5] In December 1732, the Senate and Admiralty prepared a combined document that outlined the expectations for the naval mission in the North Pacific, including specific directives for the cartographer accompanying the expedition.[6] In March 1733, the Admiralty produced its own orders that largely reiterated the earlier version, but without specifying the work the cartographer needed to complete.[7] In April, the Senate reiterated several of the previous commands, but added a requirement to investigate the current state of the China trade, an important goal in the wake of the new Treaty of Kiakhta (1727).[8]

These documents indicate a significant investment of resources from multiple government offices. Although it was clearly agreed that

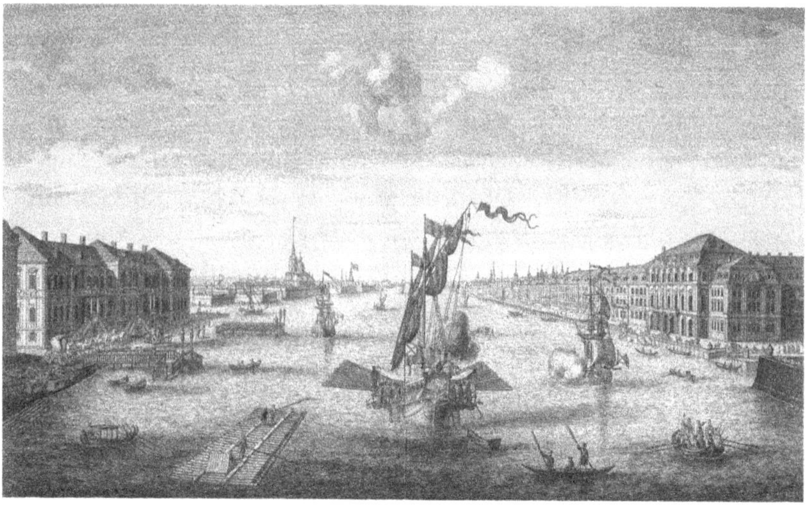

Figure 3.1. This 1750 image of St. Petersburg is centered on two key institutions, the Admiralty and the Academy of Sciences, which were joint partners on the recently concluded Second Kamchatka Expedition. "A View of St. Petersburg on either side of the River Neva, between ye Admiralty & the Academy of Sciences," The Miriam and Ira D. Wallach Division of Art, Prints and Photographs: Print Collection, The New York Public Library, New York Public Library Digital Collections, accessed June 9, 2024, https://digitalcollections.nypl.org/items/510d47db-1735-a3d9-e040-e00a18064a99.

Bering oversaw the entire production, the Senate and Admiralty had separate agendas for the expedition (figure 3.1). The expeditionary force would not travel in a single direction, nor would it depart at the same time, perhaps reflecting the multiple orders. A first group traveled north to document the coastline of the empire between Arkhangel'sk and the White Sea.[9] A second group left from Okhotsk, Russia's Pacific port, under the direction of Martin Spanberg to investigate the connection to China and Japan. A third group under Bering's personal command returned to the North Pacific to further document the coasts and resources between Kamchatka and North America. A Swedish-born naval officer, Sven Waxell, would act as Bering's second in command. This choice was more important than it might have seemed at first glance, as Bering would die from scurvy during his Pacific exploration, leaving Waxell to lead the surviving crew back to Russia.[10]

Following Bering to Okhotsk was a group of specialists, primarily physicians working as naturalists to investigate Siberia and the North Pacific. This group included Dr. Johann Georg Gmelin, who acted as the official botanist; Gerhard Friedrich Müller, who served as the historian for the expedition; and Louis Delisle de la Croyère, a rare French scientist working at the academy as a professor of astronomy.[11] Russian students from the academy also accompanied the expedition, including Stepan Krasheninnikov, who would eventually be elected as a full member to the academy in 1745 in recognition of his research during the expedition.[12] Gmelin would leave the expedition before its work was completed, and he would be replaced by another German physician acting as botanist, Georg Wilhelm Steller. Steller had married Messerschmidt's widow, who provided Steller with Messerschmidt's notes and journals. Messerschmidt's work, therefore, acted as a guidebook for this later expedition and its subsequent publications. Because Waxell, Gmelin, Müller, Krasheninnikov, and Steller would all publish accounts of the work of the expedition in Russian and German as well as in English and French, the public archive of their experiences is considerable, even without including field notes still held by the academy.[13] Their official publications were not the only discussion of the expedition in print, as its accomplishments were widely discussed across Europe in publications like the *Philosophical Transactions of the Royal Society of London*.

The personal and professional networks that supplied the academy with its specialists played a clear role in the selection of these men. Johann Georg Gmelin received his medical doctorate (MD) from the University of Tübingen in 1727 and became a member of the Russian Academy of Sciences in 1728. Upon his return from the expedition, he communicated with Linnaeus while he prepared his *Flora Sibirica*, assisting with the establishment of the Linnaeus-Russia connection that would define future scientific work inside the empire.[14] Gmelin worked as a physician and botanist in Russia until 1747, when he returned to Tübingen as a professor of medicine. His nephew Dr. Samuel Gottlieb Gmelin followed his uncle to the Russian Academy and would join the faculty at Tübingen where he finished editing *Flora Sibirica*, based on the elder Gmelin's fieldwork in Siberia during the expedition.[15] Another of Johann Georg's nephews, Dr. Johann Friedrich Gmelin, became a professor at Göttingen in 1773, where he would publish the thirteenth edition of Linnaeus's work in 1788 and 1789. The Gmelin-Linneaus network thus would continue to influence scientific productions for decades after the expedition concluded.

Whereas Gmelin arrived from one of Russia's preferred schools, Georg Wilhem Steller's recruitment followed a slightly different path. Born in Germany, he received his MD from the University of Wittenberg, which was not a typical school for Russian service. He was recruited to work as an army medic, which eventually brought him to St. Petersburg. He met Messerschmidt late in 1734, married Messerschmidt's widow in 1737, and volunteered to join the Second Kamchatka Expedition already operating in the Russian Far East. He met Gmelin in Eniseisk in 1738, who recommended Steller replace him as the naturalist for the exploration of the Kamchatkan Peninsula, where he arrived in 1740. In 1741, he accompanied Bering and his crew to Alaska and back, producing copious notes of the entire process. More famously, he had multiple disagreements with the entire crew, including Bering, Waxell, and Krasheninnikov.[16] Bering was the most frequent target of Steller's ire. As Steller later noted in his journal: "I returned with few results and useful discoveries, not through any fault of mine but because the Captain-Commander kept his promise to me so poorly that I was shown the mainland only from a distance and was finally put ashore for a few hours on three islands with great reluctance, as if I were a delinquent, without any help and with a lot of sarcastic comment in return for my honest zeal."[17] Although Steller's relationship with the officers was clearly uneasy, his educational background and knowledge of Messerschmidt's work provided a connection with the other naturalists' observations, at least in terms of the humoral rhetoric that they all employed.

The outlier of this group of German specialists was the Frenchman, Louis Delisle de la Croyère. He was recommended for the expedition by his brother, Joseph Nicholas Delisle, who was personally hired for work in Russia by Peter the Great and was among the earliest members of the academy.[18] Joseph had already established an international reputation for his accomplishments in astronomy in the 1720s.[19] In 1731, Joseph prepared cartographic information for the expedition; his brother acted as the cartographer on the expedition. After the expedition's conclusion, the work of both brothers would be questioned by its other participants, most notably Müller, who published a refutation in the 1750s. Steller was kinder in his own notes, mentioning that the "sheer ignorance" of the naval crew had led them to improperly read Delisle's map.[20] The scandal has been discussed by numerous scholars as the reaction of the academy toward those seen as critical of Russia, but it was also a reflection of the ongoing rejection of French science by Russia's Academy.[21]

The physical process of embarking on the expedition proved to be as difficult as the staffing issues. Hundreds of men, their equipment, and provisions, had to be shipped across the empire. There was an established road across Siberia, but it was a mixture of overland and river passages, highly affected by seasonal weather changes.[22] Conditions were sufficiently poor that groups of men died during the transit to Okhotsk before the expedition even began its ocean voyage in the North Pacific. For example, in 1735, almost three years after the initial guidelines were written, the main part of the expedition had reached the Siberian town of Iakutsk. One group led by Lt. Peter Lassenius, however, failed to complete their navigation of the Lena River to Iakutsk before the ice froze their vessels, forcing them to winter on "a little river not far from the mouth of the Lena. During the course of the winter they were severely ravaged by scurvy and their commander, afterwards reported that of his whole force, which had consisted of some sixty men, only three or four remained, the other having fallen." A second group, under the command of Lt. Vasilii Pronchichev, were also trapped on the west side of the river, and "were there carried off by scurvy, yet not so many of them died as to prevent the ship continuing her voyage the next year under the second-in-command. So the ship made a further attempt, but that too proved fruitless."[23] Their success rate would not improve.

Once the main part of the expedition reached Russia's Pacific port, Okhotsk, the following year, they were still in for a long wait in harsh conditions. It was necessary for the force to construct oceangoing vessels in the harbor, and then source sufficient provisions from the local environment, which proved difficult.[24] Sven Waxell, Bering's second in command, was hardly complimentary. He found Okhotsk to be "an unhealthy place, that offers no means of obtaining foodstuffs of any kind, except just in the spring, when large quantities of fish come into the river from the sea." The community needed this fish to survive the year, and therefore they salted "a large part of their catch, quantities of fish they dry in the sun or in various other ways, so that this foodstuff in more or less preserved." A primarily fish diet implied that the local community were likely phlegmatic, as the cold, moist nature of the fish would be transformed inside the body to phlegm. Although Waxell was not trained as a physician, he understood humoral theory, as the ideas transcended the scientific community to the general literate public. His conclusions on the consequences of this diet make that clear: "We observed that after our men had been eating them [fish] for several days, most of them became badly constipated and we had many cases of sickness. They can hardly be called a healthy diet. The inhabitants, however, did not become ill, presumably because they are accustomed from childhood to eat just these fish and know, so to speak, no other food."[25] The local community being adapted to their conditions and diet, whereas the new arrivals suffered from their new diet that caused putrefaction, was a conclusion that any physician might have reached.

It would not be until 1739 that the new vessels launched. Part of the fleet traveled to the Kamchatkan peninsula where they spent time investigating its coasts, settlement, and people as well as its geological features, including its volcanoes, which featured prominently in some of the published accounts of the expedition. The main part of the expeditionary force would depart from Kamchatka for North America in the summer of 1741, reaching the Alaskan coast in August. The return trip to Kamchatka was dangerous, as most of the crew had fallen ill with scurvy on the voyage. By August, the crew was dependent on scavenging resources from the islands in the North Pacific for sufficient resources in hopes of survival. Within a month, many members of the crew had died, and the survivors were shipwrecked on the island now known as Bering's Island (as Bering would die on it in December) in hopes of surviving the winter from its resources. In the spring, the few survivors, including Waxell, gathered their remaining supplies, used parts from three vessels to return one to seaworthiness, and departed for Kamchatka. Chirikov, Bering's other subordinate, was no more successful with his voyage to the Kurile Islands, because its lack of resources and food also had led to scurvy outbreak. Chirikov was sufficiently ill that command of his vessel passed to his lieutenant, but the astronomer Louis Delisle de la Croyère died from the disease during that voyage.[26] In the end, the information and materials gathered by the survivors would be sufficient evidence of the success of the expedition, but the human costs were significant.

While the expedition was ongoing, interest was growing across Europe for news of the potential discoveries. Johann Amman regularly updated Hans Sloane in London, even when the only news was an absence of information. In March 1736, for example, Amman wrote: "It is now allmost half a year that we have nothing from the Kamtschakian expedition. In their last letters they wrote, that their design was to go from Irkutskoy to Selinginsky, & from thence to Argun & Nerschkinskoy, & back again to Irkutskoy" but nothing else, including even an accurate description of where these outposts were located.[27]

Amman hoped to provide more specific details after updates from the expedition arrived in St. Petersburg two years later, but little had changed: "The professors, who undertook the journey to Kamtshatka are not arrived there as yet. On the contrary they returned last summer from Iakutsk along the river Lena to Irkutsk near the lake Baikal. About a year & half ago some vessels built at Ochotsk have put to Sea, in order to discover the Islands & Seas, wch lye between Kamtschatka, Yodso, Japan & Corea, but since that time I have heard nothing of their discoveries, or what is become of them." In fact, the hardest obstacles of the cross-Siberian journey were still to be conquered. Amman wrote:

> You may judge of the difficulty & tediousness of this undertaking from telling you, that from Iakutsk they are oblig'd to go up the Aldan, from this the Maja & Juma as far as the shallows will permit. In mounting those rivers they spend a whole summer; after wch they are obliged to carry all their baggage upon small Tega drawn by dogs, such as your manncke is, through a most desolate & cold country to Ochotsk, from whence they pass over to Kamtschatka. But in case the passage between the Island Novaia Semlia & the continent should be found most dangerous & difficult the way to Kamtschatka."[28]

Amman's final update on the expedition from 1739 hardly produced better news: "Our Kamtchkatkian Expedition gos on very slowly. The persons lead thither from the Academy have been at Irkutsk on the Lena river, but were forc'd for want of severall things to return to Irkutsk on the river Angara near the lake Baikal. Prof Muller being very much out of order, is recalled. Dr. Gmelin desires the same. There are sent allready others in their places. A Russian student is arrived in Kamtschatka." In addition to the personnel challenges, the terrain remained foreboding. He added: "The greatest difficult of this undertaking is to go from Iakutsk to Ochotsk on the Kamtschatkian Sinus. All the Country lying between those two places is the most dreadful desert. The observations of the terrible cold, of wch I wrote to you, to have been made at Olecminskoy ostrog are not made in this place, but at Kirensky Ostrog on the Lena between Irkutsk & Iakutsk not very far from the aforesaid place."[29] It is difficult to know if Amman's emphasis on the cold, barren nature of far eastern Siberia reflected the information the academy had received or was simply an excuse for a lack of information that would have sounded plausible. It was largely accurate, as the struggles with the cold environment and the difficulty of food supply were regularly mentioned in the reports that were received. Perhaps most concerning in his dispatch was the reality of experts traveling with the expedition, including Gmelin, abandoning the scientific project in favor of others, including a student (possibly Krasheninnikov) whose fieldwork would later be considered groundbreaking. This switch, however, must have raised alarms in St. Petersburg.

Interest in the expedition existed outside of the Amman-Sloane connection. Gmelin was in regular correspondence with Linnaeus, first from Siberia and then more actively once he returned to St. Petersburg, while he was completing his work on his *Flora Sibirica*. Gmelin regularly updated Linnaeus on the continuing work of the expedition from St. Petersburg, as he was in contact with Steller.[30] In the extended conversation between Gmelin and Linnaeus, Gmelin clearly accepted Linnaeus's taxonomy for plants but offered frequent corrections for classification of specific species. Linnaeus regularly advised Gmelin on his application of the system, though Gmelin moved forward with his choices, even apologizing to Linnaeus for the plants in *Flora Sibirica* that did not conform to Linnaeus's system. Gmelin accepted, however, Linnaeus's decision to sex plants, a choice Amman had rejected.[31] Although the majority of their communication involved classifying Siberian plants in Linnaeus's system, they also discussed categorizing animals, including sheep, hares, fish, and squirrels. Based on his Siberian travels, Gmelin weighed in with questions and suggestions about refining the taxonomy.[32]

For a long time, the legacy of the Second Kamchatka Expedition focused on its successes in mapping the north Pacific and the travel along the Aleutian archipelago. It was undeniably of interest across Europe, as demonstrated by a member of the Academy of Sciences publishing an explanation of Bering's success in the North Pacific to *Philosophical Transactions*.[33] After Bering's death, both the Straits and an island in that body of water were named after him in recognition of the expeditions' work. As historians and anthropologists have become more critical about Russia's colonial legacy in the north Pacific and Alaska, both in terms of the environmental damage and physical abuses of the population, the expedition became a marker of future destruction.[34] In the contemporary era, some Russian scholars have attempted to rehabilitate Russia's history in the region.[35] Ongoing work publishing and translating the records of the expedition, as well as the fieldwork conducted by men like Steller has shed new light on the remarkable contributions to botany, geology, and geography. The ethnographic legacy of the descriptions of the population produced by Gmelin and Steller, as well as the long-term effect this material had on the Russian government's view of its empire, however, need to be critically assessed.

Applying Categories

All the material produced by the expedition over the course of its operation reflects its complicated origins. It was not a single investigation but included multiple routes with multiple actors working under multiple guidelines. Personality conflicts fueled disagreements. Much of this documentation, however, described the people, geography, and climate in a similar manner, revealing how familiar humoral concepts were for these eighteenth-century figures. In terms of the scientific work of the expedition, it is arguable that Johann Georg Gmelin had the greatest impact considering the importance of his botanical work, *Flora Sibirica*, and its contribution toward Linnaeus's developing taxonomy.[36] In terms of the views of the people of the empire, Gmelin's travel narrative would be more influential. It was first published in Latin, with a German title, in four parts in 1751 and 1752, and would be translated into French within a decade.[37]

The second botanist on the expedition, Steller, would be heavily influenced by Messerschmidt's work, but Gmelin's primary reference to earlier travels in Siberia was Eberhard Isbrand Ides's embassy to China in the 1690s.[38] Unlike Steller, however, Gmelin never reviewed any of Messerschmidt's Siberian field notes, so the absence of a reference to it is quite logical.[39] Overall, Gmelin attempted to answer all the requests issued in St. Petersburg. Reflecting the instructions to the expedition from the Senate, recurring references are made to the ongoing trade with China, both to goods moving across Siberia and to local trade in different communities. Gmelin observed that textiles were the largest commodity in the trade, but other products included porcelain, tobacco, tea, sugar, sugar candy, candied ginger, and orange peel.[40] Following the first instruction from the throne, innumerable references appear to current religious practices across Siberia, with a focus on the influence that Islam held among the Tatars and those people in contact with the Central Asian khanates—including, for example, the prevalence of Persian texts among the "Muslim Tatars" of Siberia, "who are not more enlightened because of their embrace of all of these superstitions."[41] In this specific instance, Gmelin was complaining about the Tatars's confidence in Persian-language medical texts, perhaps unaware that famous works by Avicenna and Rhazes that were part of his own medical training had been written by Central Asian Muslims.

Gmelin answered the government's instructions with humoral descriptions of the people, geography, and climate and with comments on their consumption habits and religious traditions. In a sense, this was an evolution of the seventeenth-century depictions, but it also paralleled the ongoing debates about the proper classification schema for people. In Linnaeus's first edition of *Systema Naturae* (1735), he placed humankind into the new genus *Homo*, which he divided into four categories, characterized by skin color and geography: "*Europaeus albesc.* (whitish European), *Americanus rubesc.* (reddish American), *Asiaticus fuscus* (dark coloured Asian), and *Africanus nigr.* (black African)."[42] Linnaeus's categorization reflected an ongoing discussion in northern Europe that sociologist Greggor Mattson calls "ethnoracial classification," or "the measurement of population categories to inscribe the boundaries among castes, races, ethnicities, or nationalities."[43] Contemporary scholars have analyzed these human taxonomies (whether Linnaeus's or Buffon's) as the emergence of scientific racism, broadcast by Europeans globally, but whether Russia and its empire fit within this scheme was very much a question of the expedition.[44] Were Indigenous Siberians classified as European or Asian?

Linnaeus would continue to refine his system, in part by incorporating the ideas and observations of his widespread correspondents. It would not be until the tenth edition in 1759–1760, that humans became *Homo sapiens*, which remain divided into four categories primarily based on skin color, but added the importance of "physical characteristics, stature, clothing, [and] temperament, governance, and ways of living."[45] The historian Christina Skott has argued that Linnaeus's familiarity with Swedish travel narratives to Asia was a key element in his broader reassessment; however, as the historian Lisbet Koerner illustrated, Linnaeus also discussed his new idea of *Homo sapiens* with Gmelin.[46] It seems logical to assume that Gmelin's fieldwork in Siberia had some role in the changing taxonomic system.

Reading Gmelin's observations from the 1730s reveals its utility for thinking about how to categorize humankind, as he relied on what contemporary anthropologists would call "thick description" or ethnography.[47] One of the longest entries involved several groups of Tungus that he encountered, beginning outside of the Siberian town of Kuznetsk. Gmelin first spotted "several Tunguses, some in their canoes" along the bank of the Lena River; Gmelin and his compatriots "begged them to come to us, but they snuck into the forest." He encountered a second group long enough to engage them in conversation, but as he approached the group, they "retreated higher into the mountains, saying that they had nothing to give us, and that they would be ashamed to approach [the expedition] without offering presents." Despite assuring this group that the expedition intended to offer them goods, the offer "did not tempt them; as they probably took us for Slavs, who plundered these unfortunate people as soon as the opportunity arose." Although his encounter with the Tungus had not started auspiciously, Gmelin was optimistic, noting: "the women are dark and inaccessible, but they are honest; they would have wanted to talk to us, but they did not know how to speak Russian, and our Slavs who speak Tungus, only pursued conversation with the men."[48] It might be tempting to consider Gmelin's "dark" women as fitting into Linnaeus's "Asiatic" category; however, Gmelin's notes were produced at the same time Linnaeus first published. It is more likely that Gmelin relied on the humoral assessment of melancholic people having dark complexions.

Much of Gmelin's text debates his success, or lack thereof, in approaching Indigenous women across Siberia. It was a valid scientific pursuit, as the cold climate should have produced phlegmatic and melancholic men and women who struggled to procreate. The frequency of sexual encounters was, after all, a humoral nonnatural. Therefore, his ongoing investigations of the sex lives of Siberian peoples was justifiable. Among the Tungus, he noted that "the young women wear pants a little longer [than the men] but above the knee; an old habit that destroys modesty because they are very short. The women also smoke like men, and make use of Chinese tobacco; each of them had a little leather bag attached to their pants in which were tobacco, lighter, and a pipe." For Gmelin, both habits were surprising for a theoretically cold people. It was perhaps not a surprise that he invited a group of Tungus women to his boat, but only succeeded in enticing them after promising that he would provide "tobacco, flour, and bread. The contentment they felt at receiving these little presents caused us the greatest pleasure. The women wrapped the tobacco in paper, as they did with the bread and flour, and then took off their stocking and put the gifts into the other." Gmelin "recommend the women tell their husbands that they had been provided these presents," but, after waiting some time, no men came to their informal party.[49]

Even in this short summary, the humoral details are still striking. The general coloring of the Tungus and the local environment both feature in the first details. The sexual behaviors of the women are highlighted, even if it remains unclear whether Gmelin's interest was scientific or merely prurient. In this manner, he was hardly different than any eighteenth-century traveler, as the sexual habits of non-Europeans became an expected, and enticing, part of any narrative.[50] The implication may be that Gmelin and his compatriots paid these Tungus women for sexual favors, but it is far from explicitly stated. At the same time, Gmelin was adding to the expected categories of description by highlighting the features of Tungus clothing, with women in short pants here and men in finely detailed leather clothing elsewhere. Gmelin's interest in clothing may have been connected to his ongoing sexual investigation, but it also predicted Linnaeus's inclusion of clothing as a signifier in his revised taxonomy.

The details included in this description of the Tungus reflects the topics included in all the peoples described by Gmelin. The Chuvashes in European Russia, for example, "have almost all red hair. The men dress in the Russian way, but they wear short hair. Women have three dresses, but they do not think them all suitable for certain ages. The old ones wear the Russian habit. The young people have the bodice of the dress made in the Russian way, but their sleeves are made in the Polish, that is, they have an opening to pass the hands towards the middle. The lower part if hanging and is worn in a scarf."[51] Gmelin invested time and effort in noting dress styles and the cultural implications of these choices. The Chuvashes's long connection to Russia (nearly two centuries by the time of the expedition) physically appeared in the adoption of Russian dress. The distinctive aspect of the Chuvashes, their red hair, was the telltale sign of a sanguine constitution, setting them apart from the more typically melancholic and phlegmatic peoples of the empire. Sanguine people, of course, were known for their fiery temperament and sexual appetites. Chuvash women, however, seemed resistant to Gmelin's persistent attempts to see them undressed. A humoralist would consider this modesty as acting against the women's temperament, which could explain Gmelin's surprise.

A large part of Gmelin's text details differences among the many groups of Tatars he encountered, from the Volga River until far eastern Siberia. He viewed each group distinctly, as the environment was consistently shifting across the continent. Those that resided in towns were generally regarded as superior to those still living in smaller villages. The Tatars in Krasnoiarsk, for example, had "a figure that cannot displease Europeans: they have neither sunken eyes nor noses, nor a flat and wide face; they look very similar to the men of Europe. Their size is ideal; it is rare to find some that are lame or very large: they are thin, lively, laborious, affable, genuine, and sincere." The description implies that Tatars would look unfamiliar to Europeans, with sunken eyes and flat faces, and their personality should be lazy and indolent, in other words, the attitudes expected of more traditionally phlegmatic or melancholic people. Krasnoiarsk's Tatars, so active and industrious, clearly had admirable qualities: "All theft and violence are unheard of crimes among them. Libertinism and drunkenness are not common, however they are not exempt from these vices. . . . When they come into Russian towns or villages, they frequent the taverns or houses of their friend who have beer and spirits. However, it can be said in general that they are not intemperate."[52]

Gmelin often observed that the proximity to Russian communities was the common feature of the "lively, laborious" Tatars he encountered. Adopting Russian habits might improve the Tatars as well, though not to as great an extent. Among a group of Siberian Tatars in the village of Kaltirak, "fifty leagues" from the Chumysh River, a tributary of the Ob, Gmelin noted their distinct culture emerging from their environment, living "around pines, birches, and poplars" on the bank. Several of these Tatars had been baptized by the Archbishop of Tobol'sk, but Gmelin was unpersuaded that they viewed themselves as true Christians, finding no evidence of ongoing worship. However, "we came upon a Tatar woman; this woman was very beautiful, she had black hair, smooth skin, a soft, pleasant manner, and an advantageous waist." As if the details he highlighted were not sufficiently suggestive, he "asked her if she was happy with her husband, and if she did not want to have a more pleasant one. She told us that she would gladly accept this change, but that God would not want her to leave her husband." For comparison, a nearby community of Tatars to the Kaltirak village, which did not convert to Orthodoxy, had more problematic features. "These Tartars have several wives. They do not eat pork, but they drink alcohol. Their women are not beautiful, and almost all smoke tobacco."[53] Unlike his predecessors, perhaps, Gmelin had more faith in the potential for Russians to improve the qualities of their subjects. Knowing this was an official report from a state investigation, however, it may have been an acknowledgment of the expedition generating the material necessary to prove that Russian colonialism was improving Siberia, rather than failing it.

In many ways, Gmelin wrote a travel narrative that resembled the ongoing work of the broader republic of letters across Europe. Gmelin extensively detailed the history of a hermaphrodites in Siberia, once he learned that there were two in Isetskoe, a village near Tiumen', "and two more in a neighboring village: we wanted to see them. They were still childlike, and we barely distinguished what sex they belonged to; it was generally agreed they were a unique species of men. The priest of the place counted them in the ranks of men, and gave them masculine names." Gmelin gathered the four hermaphrodites and sent them for further inspection the Academy of Sciences in St. Petersburg. He did not explain if he allowed them to be accompanied on the journey, or if they, their families, or their communities consented to their removal. He did report that the academy's anatomist, who was Boerhaave's son, "proved in an undeniable way that it was indeed men," which Gmelin found surprising, as "they seemed to me to be women."[54] Dedicating a chapter to the discovery of four hermaphrodites may seem surprising considering the overall scale and variety of peoples in Siberia, but hermaphroditism was an exciting subject in the eighteenth century, especially in denoting "primitive" peoples.[55] It was simply evidence of how well the material noted by Gmelin reflected eighteenth-century interests.

Gmelin's attitudes toward Siberia's people and the characteristics with which he described them was shared by the other specialists, perhaps most by Steller, his fellow physician turned botanist. Steller shared Gmelin's reliance on humoral observations and a concern about the sexual habits and diseases of imperial subjects. For example, Steller extensively recorded the complexions of the Itelmens living on the Kamchatka peninsula. He identified them as a "mixed people. . . . Since these people could have originated from no other place than Mongolia, it follows indisputably that they emigrated to this land of Kamchatka long before the break of monarchy of the great Genghis Khan and even before the Mongols and Tungus came into being." Long exposure to the colder, and moister, environment of Kamchatka changed the Itelmens from their Mongolian origins. For Steller, the impact of the environment on physical stature was expected. As he mentioned: "Northern people are always shorter than those living in southern parts, as can be seen without extensive documentation by comparing all over the earth. Mountain people who live in valleys are always shorter than those living in broad, open regions were. People who get more physical exercise tend to be taller and stronger."[56] The Itelmens reflected this mixture of complexions, originating from a distant land, but adapted to their local environment.

Steller did not describe them as phlegmatic or melancholic, but, like Gmelin, his physical description was based in the standard images of phlegmatic or melancholic bodies. The Itelmens had a "short stature; brownish skin color; black hair; modest beards; flat faces; flattened noses; deep-set, small eyes; sparse, small eyelashes; hanging bellies; hair-free genitals; slow walk and angled steps; thin, small hands and feet; small male and large, broad female genitals; and also their timidity, fearfulness, boastfulness, timid submissiveness and stubbornness if one treats them politely." Steller's list featured the physical characteristics of a cold body: short, with small and hair-free genitals. Steller summarized his assessment with a blanket statement that the Itelmen lifestyle simply reflected their climate and diet, as expected: "Their other customs are not to be considered as much since they derive from the climate and the way in which they subsist."[57]

Much of the Itelmens' way of life confirmed Steller's diagnosis of a melancholic or phlegmatic complexion. "Generally, an Itelmen does not stir from his peace and quiet to go hunting or leave his dwelling for any reason before he is forced to do so by extreme necessity." A lack of physical activity was the primary attribute of all cold people. The Itelmens compounded this physical challenge by living on a diet of fish, which was long established to have an excess of phlegm (cold, moist complexion). Steller was compelled to mention, "no matter how much bogus proof the learned physicians maintain that fish are unhealthful, the experience of a whole nation contradicts them," because the Itelmen were prospering.[58]

Steller knew there was an essential contradiction of the Itelmens's nature. Unlike all other cold people, "these people were intent on increasing their population." In fact, unlike the majority of people living in the Russian Empire, the Itelmens "tend toward contentment and naturally, like beasts, toward lust. . . . They seek contentment in sexual pleasures. They desire to eat, drink and sleep well, and change place and company often in order not to become ill-humored. They seek frequent sexual intercourse with different partners and fantasize voluptuously, maintaining and inciting these fantasies by dancing, singing, and by telling entertaining stories."[59] For Steller, the Itelmens's mixed character produced an unexpected outcome—a cold people who were interested in sex.

Steller presents the sex lives and marriage habits of the Itelmens in great detail, describing different- and same-sex sexual encounters for both sexes as an ordinary part of life. "Nonetheless, the men are not jealous, living on the sly with many other women and young girls, which they like a lot, but the men have to guard their secret carefully because their women are very jealous, although the latter demand freedom in everything, covet the love of other men, and are insatiable and above all so conceited that she who can list the most lovers is considered the happiest woman, and they try to outdo each other in bragging." He added in a note that "women also commit adultery with women, by way of the clitoris . . . These people also have male lovers whom the men, in addition to their wives, make use of through the posterior without any jealousy. In the past, the women also committed sodomy with dogs a lot."[60]

Although the mixed physical qualities offered a potential idea why the Itelmens were sexualized, Steller offered another reason: "What makes these people so lecherous and prone to venery is probably the consumption of so many fish eggs and bulbs, as well as moldy fish—their winter food turning completely moldy, sharp and acrid—for semen is frequently generated and the blood vessels are stimulated by the stinking fish fat." As proof of this theory, Steller "experimented" on an Itelmen woman "who ate at my table for a half a year and was totally kept from the usual food became much more moderate and modest."[61]

Although Steller began his description of the Itelmens noting their large population, he believed that "the Itelmen in marriage are more intent on sexual pleasure than procreation and increasing their families, which can be concluded from the fact that they prevent pregnancy by various medicines and that they seek to abort by means of herbs as well as violent external means. They also used to expose the newborn children in the manner of the old Germans or even to strangle them with their own hands, which still happens today now and then." In addition, later in his notes Steller mentioned a "decoction of wild celery," which men used to treat scurvy and women to prevent pregnancy, but he offered no comments on its effectiveness. He mentioned, however, that the local cure for venereal disease was a "decoction of the beautiful yellow-flowered leatherleaf," but it was not a success.[62]

Steller's account might reflect his own sexual interests more than the reality of life among the Itelmens in the early eighteenth century. Steller's physical description of a typical Itelmen with small, hair-free genitals suggests some familiarity with their bodies, and his comment that they sought intercourse through dancing and singing suggests that he, not necessarily the objects of his observation, found this material enticing. He also mentions that anyone who lives on Kamchatka must "acquire a woman or live in secret understanding with another's wife" from "necessity," because "no one washes or sews for him, takes care of him or does him any favors unless he pays with sexual intercourse."[63] Regardless of the morality of the situation, Steller's objectification of the Itelemens is striking. The people of Kamchatka were objects for experimentation for him.

Steller's discussion of sexual activity reflected a growing anxiety around the empire's sexual habits and its potential effects on population growth.[64] For Russia, the Second Kamchatka Expedition only fueled this anxiety with the realization that Russia was filled with a variety of physical body types: could there be one solution for the procreation challenge? In this way, Steller's contribution, while exploitative, contributed toward the pursuit of a solution to the empire's greatest challenge. There may be no evidence indicating moldy fish was prescribed as a new type of aphrodisiac following the expedition, but Steller's work presented the idea that local cures for Russian problems could be discovered. At the same time, Steller's observations on the widespread venereal epidemic on the Kamchatkan peninsula only highlighted a growing health crisis for which no one in the empire yet had a successful solution. More sex could be better, but not if it produced more disease. Russia's management of its empire was a mixed success at best.

Steller's unpublished notes highlighted the ways in which the members of the expedition documented Russia's ongoing challenges in managing its empire. Endemic diseases, including venereal conditions, threatened Russia's ability to populate its territory. Published records from the expedition, like Gmelin's, could have been read in similar ways, but, at the time, his unique ethnographic descriptions of the peoples of Siberia fueled the ongoing taxonomic project of eighteenth-century Europe. Although the Linnaean system was not the only option in the 1730s and 1740s, Linnaeus's connection with the Russian scientific establishment predated the work the expedition and would continue for decades to come. The type of information Gmelin noted as having significance for understanding body types—including clothing and lifestyle—would be included in Linnaeus's later edition of his *Systema Naturae*. Clearly, the ongoing work in Russia reflected a broader European process of categorizing humankind. The unanswered question of the Second Kamchatka Expedition would occupy Russia's naturalists for decades to come: were Indigenous Siberians European or Asian? Most were phlegmatic or melancholic, but their mixed European-Asian features had yet to be placed in the new taxonomic system.

Managing Scurvy

Although the attention of Europe's naturalists may have been focused on the information unearthed by the Second Kamchatka Expedition, the discoveries from Siberia and the North Pacific did little, if anything, to alter the concerns about the danger of Russia's climate. As Gmelin corresponded with Linnaeus to debate classification, British diplomats loudly protested the dangerous climate in European Russia, long considered more temperate than Siberia's extremes. Claudius Rondeau, the British consul during the 1730s, regularly described the ongoing stress of life in Russia—its extremely cold winters and its hot and dry summers sparking fires that left "every body here in the greatest terrour and consternation."[65]

If the climate was not sufficiently challenging, the return of the plague in 1738 was perhaps too much for Rondeau. The plague spread along Russia's border with Poland-Lithuania, thought to be the outcome of Poland's current war with the Ottoman Empire. The Russian government had imposed quarantines along the border as soon as the news arrived, but "the plague had broke their measures" by September 1738.[66] Rondeau mentioned that it was well known that the plague was endemic to Ukraine, and therefore it was impossible to campaign in the region without risking exposure.[67] By December, the government enacted a series of quarantine lines between the front and the Russian heartland. The new measures seemed effective, as "no body was permitted to come from the Army to Mosco, without doing Quarantine at twenty verst from that Citty, or bringing a Passport from the Felt Marshall Munick or some other General Officer. I have even been assur'd, that the Plague was actually got into some few houses in the Ukraine, but by burning them, it's at present intirely ceased."[68] Although quarantines and fires were used as the state's best defenses. Rondeau understood the operation of the plague in accordance with conventional wisdom of that era. To him, the public health measures could control the plague, but the climate ultimately won. "It's report'd here as certain, that there is nothing to be fear'd from the Plague, tho' it was some time ago on the Borders of the Ukraine & even in a little Village near Carkoff. This Ministry assures it is intirely stop'd, & if any infections should yet remain in those Distant parts, the excessive Cold Weather, we have had for some Weeks, will infallibly drive it away & purify the Air."[69] For Rondeau, the cold's ability to mitigate the spread of the plague was a benefit to Russia. The climate offered protection from the ongoing danger of southern entanglements in the Ottoman Empire.[70] Rondeau was not a physician, but the ability of cold weather to defeat the plague was established medical knowledge, a part of Sydenham's nosology, among other proponents.[71]

Even if the plague was defeated by Russia's climate, the British complexion was not suited toward the cold. Rondeau had complained for a decade about his poor health from St. Petersburg's climate. In September 1739, when Rondeau wrote to the foreign secretary in London with apologies for having "been so very ill, My Lord, for ten days past occasioned by a great cold, which we often get in this hard climate."[72] Unlike his previous illnesses, this one would prove fatal a week later.[73] Rondeau's illness was quite painful, according to an account provided by his nephew. It began with "a Diarrhea that lasted thirteen Days, and then suddenly turned to a nervous feavour and defluxion upon his Breast with a continual delirium until his Death."[74] From the symptoms, it is not clear what this illness may have been, but it is clear it was not a simple cold. In Rondeau's correspondence, the cold climate may have saved the Russian Empire from a plague outbreak in 1738, but it was also the climate that ultimately destroyed his health and took his life.

Rondeau marked the beginning of a long line of British diplomats who connected Russia's climate to their poor health in St. Petersburg. John Carmichael, the Earl of Hyndford, was another. In January 1749, he protested to the foreign secretary that he was "in pain for the rest of my Equipage & my provisions" because "after nine days of the Strongest Frost that ever was known in Russia, there has been such a Thaw during fourteen days consecutively, that all the roads & most of the rivers are quite broke up, a thing never yet known in this Country," making it impossible for his baggage to be delivered to St. Petersburg upon his arrival.[75] Less than a month later, Carmichael submitted a request to the foreign secretary to receive permission to leave Russia for spas in Germany. He hoped to be relieved of his office early enough to reach his destination before the season was over to avoid "the great Detriment to my health."[76] The long delay in perceiving permission caused a minor crisis for Carmichael, who not only missed the spa season but also was prevented by his illness from attendance at court. When questioned by the Russian minister, Aleksei Petrovich Bestuzhev-Riumin, why he desired such a rapid departure from the court, Hyndford could not help but reveal that it was "on account of his Health." As proof, Carmichael "shew'd Him my Hands, that are full of Scurvy Spots. Therefore, it was necessary to access "the Air, and of making Use of Mineral Waters" in Germany, as the only solution to mitigate the damage of living "in this cold Climate."[77]

Carmichael was the first British diplomat to suggest that scurvy was a natural outcome of the cold climate, but this association—between scurvy and Russia's climate—had been well established in medical circles. The Second Kamchatka Expedition had been plagued by the disease, and it was known to have caused both Bering and Deslisle's deaths, among others. It would have very much been on the mind of the court in the 1740s. As a result of this interest, the naturalists of the academy investigated all potential cures across the empire as scurvy was a persistent endemic challenge.[78] A cure for scurvy, or at least a successful treatment regimen, would bring fame and recognition to the academy for its work and would facilitate Russian colonization and settlement not only in Siberia but also North America.

It was not until the 1920s that vitamin C was discovered. Although modern physicians know scurvy is a vitamin C deficiency, historical "scurvy" was an amalgamation of symptoms before the twentieth century, the cause of which was widely debated.[79] Weakness and fatigue were regularly noted but could have applied to a myriad of diseases. The pathognomonic symptom for scurvy was bleeding gums, but now we know that is also a sign of an advanced case. Scurvy commonly afflicted sailors, but their diet was so poor, primarily consisting of water, dried beef, and desiccated bread (so-called biscuit), any number of nutritional diseases could have affected them. Before vitamins, therefore, scurvy was a broad category to describe any illness at sea.

Further complicating a diagnosis for scurvy, much less a treatment, was that physicians were quite certain that scurvy existed in two separate forms: land scurvy and sea scurvy. The symptoms were similar, but the causes were distinct. In the seventeenth century, sea scurvy was caused by long exposure to moist, cold air. Some argued that long-term separation from the land was unnatural, and only a reconnection to soil could solve this type of "earthsickness," as historian Joyce Chaplin termed it.[80] This inspired the habit among crews of eating as many green plants as possible upon returning to shore; it was a means of reconnecting to the land. Cynical modern scholars might suggest that greens were a significant improvement of the diet of sailors. They might not have contained vitamin C (some do of course), but vegetable matter in general could address other nutritional imbalances in the body. Whereas sea scurvy was caused by excess cold, making its occurrence over water common, land scurvy was attributed to hot causes, including acidic foods. The reason was its association with the initial symptoms of pimples and ulcers, signs of excess heat in the body. Patients suffering from land scurvy could be bled to reduce the heat, or given cooling foods, particularly white foods that were known to produce phlegm in the body.[81]

Both Steller and Waxell produced detailed accounts of managing scurvy among the crew during the Pacific voyage. Steller regularly encouraged the crew to consume as many greens as possible, whereas Waxell endorsed traditional naval solutions, including fresh air and hard work.[82] Waxell's narrative is by far the most thorough on the scurvy outbreak, perhaps as a result of his official responsibilities in evaluating the expedition. Both Waxell and Steller shared the opinion that the scurvy facing the crew was a result of putrefaction of the humors in the body. As the cold closed the pores, humors accumulated leading to rot, which was clearly diagnosable by the bad breadth of the sailors. According to Waxell, the problems began for the crew in Okhotsk before their departure, as the only food available was salted fish, resulting in constipation among the crew, an obvious step toward putrefaction. As much as salt was considered to be a cause of scurvy, constipation was known to be one of its first symptoms. Following a spring departure in 1741, Waxell recorded that scurvy had spread among the entire crew by August, which he believed was induced by the lack of fresh provisions and clean water. A storm drove their ship ashore in October, with the crew landing on an island they would name for Bering following his death in December.The climate of the island exacerbated their condition, according to Waxell, from its "continuing dampness," and the lack of food and gin only worsened their condition. Gin, in particular, had kept the men "in a fairly good fettle." Throughout October and November, "there were few who were still on their feet . . ., and so reluctant to do any work. . . . Their only wish, indeed, was that a speedy death might free them from their miserable plight."[83] Gin may not have been a traditional remedy, but as Waxell was convinced that melancholy was one of the most dangerous symptoms, and it, apparently, was best treated with alcohol.[84]

Beyond his unconventional ideas of treatment, Waxell held many traditional views of the dangers of scurvy. When the boat shipwrecked, most of the crew moved to the shore, but Waxell avoided this for as long as possible. He observed that "Many died on deck as soon as they were brought out into the air," a longstanding belief that a change in air quality could produce rapid death. To avoid this fate, he attempted to stay in his quarters on board, keeping himself warm with a small fire. However, "the bad air and filth found its way even there from the holds where so many had been lying ill for two or even three months, attending to the needs of nature where they lay. I suffered so severely from this evil, unhealthy stench that I became unable to use either my feet, hands, or my teeth, and so was as good as ready to be claimed by death." As a result, the able-bodied among the crew decided to move Waxell off the ship, though he was careful to take the precaution of wrapping his whole face in a "thick warm cap and placed another on his head" so fearful was he of the possibility of dying from exposure to clean air.[85]

Although dozens of sailors would die on Bering's Island, including Bering, Waxell and a skeleton crew would slowly regain their health over the winter and launch a rebuilt ship in the spring to return to Kamchatka. Waxell paid extensive attention to the varieties of meat the crew consumed over the winter, as fresh food was necessary for recovery. He ranked young sea-lions "as the best eating of all," sea-bear flesh as "revolting, because it has a very strong and unpleasant smell, more or less like that of an old goat," and a dead whale as "rank" but nonetheless as "a good fortune." Despite his interest in describing the new meats available from the local waters, Waxell concluded that "the green shoots," collected by their botanist, Steller, made the greatest difference. They used "some for drinking, some for eating, and by taking them we found our health noticeably improved." He concluded, "from my own experience I can assert that none of us became well or recovered his strength completely before we began eating something green, whether plant or root."[86]

Waxell's observations on the disease differ slightly from the records of both Steller and Gmelin. Gmelin addressed the disease as he did all illnesses in expedition, first describing the symptoms and then the treatment. He wrote: "The symptoms of scurvy were pains residing in places where we had injuries or abscesses, fatigue accompanied by extraordinary slumber, swelling of the feet on which appeared here and there blue spots, a violent sneezing which caused an incredible pain in the kidneys, sore teeth, foul breath, swelling throughout the body accompanied by an unquenchable thirst, a dry cough, and a kind of constipation, the effects of which lasted two or three weeks, and the most powerful purgatives were without effect." The cure he outlined was one that would have been familiar to many—avoiding excessive cold, taking in as much fresh air as possible to "drive out the harmful vapors," and hard work. In fact, more than four hours of sleep a day was to be avoided.[87]

Gmelin, however, departed the expedition before the North Pacific journey, ceding his role as botanist to Steller. Therefore Steller had an opportunity to add to Gmelin's Siberian observations with his fieldwork in Kamchatka and North America. The Itelmen, for example, "easily cure scurvy with frozen fish in the winter and with fresh fish, garlic, and other herbs in the summer."[88] After their voyage, his official narrative recorded a commitment to eating fresh herbs and berries and drinking spring water as the most effective treatment. According to Steller, the crew's rejection of his advice ultimately led to the deadly outbreak.

At several stops, he urged the crew to load as much clean water (avoiding the salt or lime deposits along the shore) and fresh plants as possible, but to no avail. Leaving Shumagin Island, for example, he asked the men "to gather up as many antiscorbutic plants as we would need, [but] the gentlemen scorned even this proposal, so valuable to themselves and for which they should have thanked me."[89] Therefore, when they fell ill, Steller concluded that it was their fault, his criticism reflecting his personality conflicts with the crew.

Steller's prophylactic treatment for himself proved successful, as he was one of the few able-bodied men when the crew landed on Bering's Island. There he would spend time hunting for herbs and greens rather than hunting sea-cows and sea-otters, which Waxell would later record in great detail. There was no doubt to Steller that his gathering was the key to the crew's cure. In the spring, "we also got many edible and tasty plants and roots; eating these provided variety as well as medicine for our emaciated bodies." The plants included sweet grass, bitter cress, brookline, figwort, and lingonberries.[90]

Steller, Gmelin, and Waxell might have disagreed on treatment, but the one issue that no one in the crew challenged was the cause of the disease. Waxell summarized their conclusions in a chapter on scurvy at the end of his narrative: "Its cause is presumably to be found in the continual diet of salt and dry foods and in the often stinking and putrid water on which they must subsist. [The crew] work hard and so become exhausted, while the continual damp raw weather may also play its part." As the crew became tired, their depression would transition to the disease's second stage, in which visible symptoms, including bleeding gums and swollen limbs, and constipation occurred.[91]

Scurvy not only was a problem for Russia's exploration of its empire nor its future settlement but also was an increasing concern of all ocean-going European empires in the eighteenth century. Contemporary physicians across Europe were studying outbreaks and developing new therapies in hopes of alleviating the condition. The best known of these men was the British physician, James Lind, who published the first edition of his groundbreaking study, *A Treatise of Scurvy*, in 1753. The challenge was obvious, physicians had "ascribed to this modern calamity" a "very extraordinary number of scorbutic symptoms." Despite more than a century of investigation, Europe was still plagued by "the inefficacy of one uniform method of cure." The "simple antiscorbutics" being proscribed "failed to remove the many various and complicated disorders that were classed under the name scurvy."[92] Considering the clear association of the Russian Empire and scurvy following the

Second Kamchatka Expedition, it should not be surprising that Lind turned to his professional contacts working in the Russian Empire for the latest information about scurvy before publishing his study.

Lind's Russian informant was John Cook, a Scottish doctor in Russian service, who arrived in Russia from Scotland in 1735 and worked for the navy in Kronstadt, Azov, Astrakhan, and Riga. Cook's information had arrived late in the production process for Lind's treatise but were included as Lind felt the information was too significant to leave out. Cook sent Lind his notes on several Russian scurvy outbreaks, beginning with Azov. To set the scene, Cook described the environment of Azov in some detail, including that it was "situated, as most towns on the banks of that river [the Don], on a low sandy soil, and surrounded with lakes, marshes, and woods. The winter commonly begins in the month of October. In November, all the rivers, lakes, and marshes are quite frozen over, and the whole country is covered with snow; which continues until about the beginning of April." In other words, Azov certainly had a cold and moist climate. While serving there in the winter of 1739, "scurvy made its appearance" in February, but the peasants "were not so much afflicted with it as the sailors, nor the sailors so much as the soldiers. Many, both sailors and soldiers, were sent to our hospital"; most of the patients were discharged by April. Cook's argument was that the labor each group exerted played a role in the severity of their illness, as the peasants provided heavy labor all winter, and the sailors remained involved in shipbuilding, leading to fewer cases. Soldiers, wintering in the barracks, suffered the highest incident rate. Astrakhan provided a similar case study, with a moist location "on small island washed by the Volga." Cook added: "The garrison soldiers are much more subject to the scurvy than the boors [serfs], and these last than the sailors. The soldiers live a very indolent life, having but little duty to perform. They eat hardly any thing else, even in their hospitals, besides rye break and meal, with fish; and have nothing but water for drink. . . . The hospitals are very damp and rotten." Sailors, by comparison, "work hard at all times of the year, both in the docks and at sea; and live much better, having good provisions of all sorts."[93] It is not difficult to understand the appeal of Cook's case notes for Lind, as hard labor as the most reliable cure for scurvy had long been a guiding principle of the British navy.

Of the outbreaks Cook discussed, the Riga outbreak in 1751 within the local garrison was the most severe. Cook remembered it as the "most dreadful spectacle" that he ever witnessed. "Their rotten gums gangrened, as also their lips, which dropped off; the sphacelus spread to the cheeks, and muscles of their lower jaw; and the jaw-bone in some fell down upon the sternum. . . . Nothing but death rid the unhappy wretches of their frightful misery." At Riga, Cook applied the therapeutic treatment "practiced in Russia, especially by the German physicians and surgeons" for "hot or painful scurvy." It began with a "very gentle purge or two," followed by a mixture of antiscorbutics, then "fresh flesh-meat every day, and what greens or salads we could procure them. They used the warm bath once or twice a-week." Finally, Cook "obliged them to use exercise, and to walk about both forenoon and afternoon, when the weather would permit. I allowed them to sleep moderately; and forbid them all dried, salt, and fat meats. Fumigating the wards, is common in all the hospitals in Russia."[94] The Riga case was the one in which Cook offered new ideas for the treatment of scurvy. While identifying this scurvy outbreak as hot (i.e., land scurvy), he implemented a regimen that had been developed at sea, including the diet, exercise, and clean air. Without question, his successful treatments in Riga supported Lind's argument that only a single scurvy existed, and not different diseases hiding under a single name.

After his service in Russia, Cook published a narrative of his experiences at work in the country. Unsurprisingly, he discussed his work on scurvy as his most important accomplishment while in Russia, noting the value of his work to Lind in the 1750s. Published in 1770, more than two decades after the outbreaks in Azov or Astrakhan, Cook's assessment of the best therapeutic strategy had not evolved. A poor diet and lack of exercise remained the primary causes of scurvy. Cook described that when he "saw what dismal havock this disease would make in the garrison, I regretted the want of gardens, where fresh herbs, and excellent vegetables might have been nursed up for the use of the sick." Unfortunately, "these gardens were at the time dressed up for the use of the colonels, lieutenant-colonels, and majors, and the hospitals for which they were designed had not the smallest use of them." Cook added further incidents of scurvy in this later narrative, including an early episode in 1744, just after arriving in Russia. He treated a young boy in Moscow, who suffered from a "scorbutic cough," not known as a traditional symptom of scurvy. Cook argued that an earlier doctor had misdiagnosed the cough as a sign of consumption. Cook's regimen of fresh air and light in the boy's bedroom, and a course of light exercise, along with "proper medicines in a few weeks, recovered him to his former state of health."[95] It is certainly possible that Cook's narrative was an attempt to gain further notice as an expert on scurvy, as he pushed the boundaries of what the disease was known to be. In this instance, his scurvy therapy resolved a cough; an argument for its value as a practice.

Although Cook sought relevance outside of Russia after his departure from the empire, he had been a significant figure in the Russian medical establishment during his time in service. Before his postings to the military hospitals in Azov, Astrakhan, and Riga, he had been an instructor for military surgeons in St. Petersburg. His scurvy therapeutic regimen was a part of Russian medical practice.[96] It was not as innovative as he might have preferred for his personal fame, as none of his treatments had not been tried as part of the Second Kamchatka Expedition's search for a cure for scurvy. In his original notes to Lind, Cook confessed he was simply applying the lessons of the "Germanic physicians" working in the country, which included both Gmelin and Steller. Although there was no direct path from their work to Lind's treatise, there was an informal path through the British medical practitioners like Cook sharing these methods.

The middle of the eighteenth century was a pivotal moment for scurvy intervention, particularly for the British Empire during and after the Seven Years' War with its acquisition of Canada.[97] Lind may have been concerned about the fate of the British navy, but Russia's officers were no less concerned about the health of their troops. Waxell implemented every possible solution to try to preserve his crew in the north Pacific and reported this information to the Admiralty as part of this duties. Russia's army officers faced similar struggles. C. H. von Manstein, a foreign officer in military service, published a narrative of his experiences with the army during the war with the Ottoman Empire that began in 1736. His troops were plagued by a general fatigue created by "incessant marches." He concluded, "notwithstanding all that has been said of the Russians and their being so robust and hardy, they are subject to several diseases, as the scurvy and fevers, also in the field to dysentery." The death toll from the regular scurvy outbreaks in the army could be as high as one-third.[98] Cook argued that the garrison troops' lack of exercise was a root cause of the likelihood of suffering from scurvy, but Manstein argued that overwork and a poor diet produced the same results among those same troops. Manstein was also serving before the Second Kamchatka Expedition departed Okhotsk for North America. It is possible that the state of medical knowledge changed in the wake of the return of the expedition, but it is also possible that officers were not as current about disease studies as a physician such as

Cook would have been. It may also have been that it was easier for a foreign specialist like Lind to accept Cook's Russian information because it aligned with his assessment of the disease. Confirmation bias is not a new phenomenon, after all. In either case, the state of medical knowledge in Russia was current compared with studies across Europe. These physicians were in regular contact with one another. The challenge for Russia was no different than that in other countries—disseminating the latest information to improve the health of the empire.

While the Second Kamchatka Expedition was an ongoing concern, the Academy of Sciences and the College of Medicine made decided attempts to improve the health of the empire. Cook reflected the general improvement of the health of the military forces, as they developed an active process of recruiting foreign doctors and having them not only serve in military hospitals and with the troops but also train Russian surgeons for duty. His correspondence network brought Russian-generated knowledge out to the wider medical community and provided a route for new information and therapies to arrive and be deployed among the military. The academy was no less concerned, as it produced a large compendium of information, the *Florinova ekonomiia* in 1738. It was the first publication produced in Russia that included specific guidance on treating "the French disease," at the same moment Steller was observing the damage that had been done by venereal diseases in Kamchakta. According to the manual, the disease "comes from visiting dishonest and impure places" (*nechestnykh i nechistnykh mest*). The signs of the infection became visible on the body, with excessive heat and restless sleeping, a pale or yellow color for the skin, red stains on the forehead, and sores on the mouth. The academy's recommendation was either a preparation relying on mercury, or a syrup infused with sassafras. Although the original version of the text was published in German by the academy in 1738, which was logical for the extensive staff of Germans working at the academy, the text was published in a Russian translation in 1760 to increase its accessibility.[99] If the expedition was most successful at demonstrating how complex the population of the Russian Empire was, then the academy was already implementing steps, albeit small ones, to improve health.

The expedition and its work on scurvy was not the only attempt to challenge the criticism of Russia's climate. In the fall of 1739, the Academy of Sciences developed plans to transform the traditional icehouse placed on the Neva River in St. Petersburg with a far more grandiose

"Ice Palace" the following winter. The entire enterprise would be documented, including the detailed blueprints of the ambitious construction made of ice, placed on the ice, for the court's entertainment. As the academy's pamphlet on the palace explained, "Ice has hitherto been regarded as a kind of material in which art can only exert little or no effort," and the ice palace revealed the beautiful "fluidity of water" thanks to the craftsmanship of Russia's artists.[100] The publication by the Academy of Sciences, including the plentiful images, was a strategy to promote Russia's mastery of the winter across Europe. It is hard to say whether it achieved this goal. Britain's diplomats, among the most consistent critics, never once mentioned its construction or the subsequent balls held in its structure.

Physicians and naturalists who spent time in Russia noted its climate was extreme, both hot and cold, and both conditions risked the health of its residents. Humoralism expected temperate balance as the ideal state; any extreme change to one of the nonnaturals (climate, food, or exertion) would be dangerous. Cold caused the putrefaction of the humors inside the body, and, without the ability to manage this condition, illnesses resulted. This knowledge was so widely accepted that these conditions were exploited not only by men such as the British diplomats at the start of the eighteenth century but also by physicians writing in London with only a secondhand knowledge of Russia. The early steps for the Russian medical establishment to apply their knowledge to the empire's health challenges had only begun to be recognized by foreign experts like Linnaeus and Lind.

These small steps were followed by others. In 1760, for example, the Royal Society for the Arts, Manufactures, and Commerce in London debated a recommendation from one its members, as it sought a solution for a successful feed crop for cattle "in those northern Countries." Working alongside "Mr Kalm . . . who had been a disciple of Doctor Linnaeus," they gathered seeds of various grasses from Canada and Siberia and ran a trial in both Sweden and Britain to see if a successful cold crop could be cultivated. The best result of this experiment was "Gennial Vetch from Siberia" (*Vicia sativa*), which thrived for two years, but "the Cold of the last winter killed all the plants."[101] The failure of that trial raised questions about this botanical knowledge extracted from Siberia, but the fact that the British looked to Russia for potential solutions was a sign of Russia's physicians' and naturalists' role as producers of knowledge.

Chapter 4

Improving Health, Inoculating Smallpox

The Second Kamchatka Expedition was a remarkable achievement for the state. Its publications, including Johann Georg Gmelin's *Flora Sibirica*, demonstrated the wealth of resources that the Russian Empire contained. New maps of Russia's Pacific coastline and northwest America documented its enormous territorial reach. The scientific merit of the expedition, particularly the work of its cartographer, Louis Delisle de la Croyère, remained under debate. Delisle's observation that Siberia was so cold that the mercury is his thermometer had frozen raised several questions, leading the academy's scientists to replicate his experiment in St. Petersburg two decades later.[1] Much of the interest in Europe, however, remained focused on the ethnographic material published, which revealed as many concerns about Russia's empire as its successes. These texts described the empire's territory as underpopulated, if not occupied by melancholic and phlegmatic people, who lacked the industry or energy to maximize the benefits of Russia's material bounty. The search for local remedies to overcome these unsuitable bodies was ongoing, but, by the expedition's conclusion, that quest was still a work in progress. This is not to suggest that the ethnographic material produced by the expedition was not well received. It provided new data for Carl Linnaeus's taxonomy, and the types of material gathered reflected the reformed system that Linnaeus first suggested in the tenth edition of his *Systema Naturae* (1759–1760). In fact, Linnaeus justified Gmelin's fascination in the 1730s with clothing and lifestyle when Linnaeus added those features in his revised taxonomy.

With physicians in prominent roles in the expedition, it is not a surprise that the data they gathered also contributed to medical science, in particular, to the treatment of two of Russia's endemic diseases, scurvy and syphilis. The work of Gmelin and Georg Wilhelm Steller also highlighted that some diseases, especially smallpox, were uncontrolled. Smallpox's devastating consequences for the population, particularly in Siberia, was a consistent source of criticism throughout the eighteenth century, to which Gmelin and Steller may have unintentionally contributed. The concern did not begin with the expedition, as Philipp Johann von Strahlenberg was among those who blamed Russian colonial settlement for infecting Siberians. As he wrote, "Pox, (Small) was formerly unknown to the *Pagan Koraeiki*, *Lamuti*, and *Kamtschadali*, about the Bay of Lama. But since the Russians have got Possession of those Countries, these Pagans have received the Infection from them, and great Numbers dy[e] of this Distemper."[2] Anyone reading a narrative about travel or exploration across the Russian Empire would have encountered similar claims.

Undoubtedly, this was a balancing act. Promoting the scientific work of Russia's physicians positioned the empire in the center of scientific debates across Europe, but publishing observations about the underpopulation of Siberia and the state's inability to intervene in the health of the public provided ample evidence for the state's critics. Eighteenth-century writers were increasingly concerned with population size as the signpost for a successful state. Public debates about population size and the promotion of gynecology and obstetrics were occurring across Europe.[3] Although the Russian Empire was no different in this regard, the published narratives highlighting Siberia's empty spaces undermined its other efforts.[4] As French critics of the empire became increasingly public in their attacks on the Russian Empire in general and on Catherine the Great (r. 1762–1796) in particular, the Russian government focused on increasing the population, not only through natalist policies but also with health interventions to control its endemic diseases. The culmination of this intentional turn was a widespread inoculation program to prevent smallpox, which was adopted earlier than in most European states. Rather than the government being overwhelmed by the complexity and scale of the empire, Russia's launch of one of the most expansive inoculation programs proved to be an innovative success.[5]

Climate Critics

One aspect of the ongoing investigations of climate in the eighteenth century involved a theory promoted by some Enlightenment thinkers now called "climate determinism." This idea suggested that climate influenced not only the constitution of bodies and overall health but also the culture of those people, particularly their political development.[6] For some French *philosophes*, Russia served as the ideal model of political development in a cold climate. Siberia's underpopulation and the empire's undeveloped resources provided evidence of the ineffectiveness of the Russian government. An intemperate climate produced an intemperate government, which failed to effectively improve the empire.

The most well-known climate determinist in the eighteenth century was Baron de Montesquieu, who critiqued Russia's climate and its government in *The Spirit of Law* (1748).[7] In his view, Russia's cold produced not only its autocracy but also its negative social and cultural consequences. He wrote: "The strength of the fibres in northern nations is the cause that the coarsest juices are extracted from their ailments. From hence two things result: one that the parts of the chyle or lymph are more proper, by reason of their large surface, to the applied to, and to nourish, the fibres: the other, that they are less proper, because of their coarseness, to give a certain subtilty to the nervous juice. Those people have therefore large bodies and little vivacity."[8] A nation populated by peoples of little vivacity had been the long-term problem confronting Russia. Warmer climates had always been associated with energy and industry; cold climates produced laziness. According to Montesquieu, cold countries also had "little sensibility for pleasure," which was the source of their ongoing population challenge.[9]

Aside from the reliance on old tropes of cold bodies, Montesquieu added new details to the implicit challenge of life in the north. Alcohol was necessary for survival: "In cold countries the aqueous part of the blood is very little evacuated by perspiration. They make therefore make use of spirituous liquors, without which the blood would congeal. They are full of humours; consequently strong liquors, which give a motion to the blood, are proper for those countries." It followed logically that people in hot climates should not drink alcohol, which is why the Muslims in the Middle East abstained. However, "Such a law would be improper for cold countries, where the climate seems to force them to a kind of national drunkenness, very different from personal intemperance. Drunkenness predominates over all the world, in proportion to the coldness and humidity of the climate."[10]

Montesquieu did not offer the only perspective on Russia's challenges during the Enlightenment. Nor was he the only *philosophe* focused on the problematic government of Russia, given that any intemperate region suffered from some lack in comparison to temperate Europe. Events in Russia, however, soon proved that Montesquieu's criticism of the empire was justified. Hardly a decade after Montesquieu depicted Russia as an empire of "national drunkenness" and "little vivacity," Tsar Peter III (r. 1762-1763) was overthrown by his wife, Catherine, giving French critics an opportunity to depict the lack of effective leadership in Russia. Claude-Carloman de Rulhière, a young French diplomat in Russia in 1762, wrote a description of Catherine's illegal rise to power. Catherine intervened to prevent the text's publication until after her death, fearing damage to her reputation abroad.[11] Russia's ongoing problems were obvious to Rulhière. Once Peter became tsar, he "began his reign by an edict, whereby, in the plentitude of his arbitrary power, he granted to the Russian nobility the rights of a free nation; and as if, in reality, the rights of the people depended upon the concession, the edict produced such violent transports of joy, that this vain nation proposed to erect from him a statue of massy gold." It was clear that Russia was unprepared to be a modern nation. Catherine and Nikita Ivanovich Panin, who Rulhière considered to be Catherine's primary ally, were "united in the resolution of rescuing their country from despotism."[12] Rulhière also described at length Catherine's reliance on military force to manage a coup and execute her husband.

Rulhière's depiction of Russia confirmed Montesquieu's argument on the consequences of the climate. Its people were confused by basic concepts of political authority, leading them to accept a government based in despotic control. Peter III accomplished sweeping reforms—but only when implemented by foreigners, who also turned the court into a hotbed of sexual politics. For Rulhière, both sex and politics were foreign accomplishments. The changing medical ideas—the emergence of a neo-Hippocratic tradition—may have been unknown to the general public. Montesquieu's view of the government and its connection to the climatic conditions may have been better known among Europe's educated elite. But Catherine's coup proved Montesquieu's criticism was correct—that the climate created a dangerous country—and Rulhiére offered the proof.

French critics of Russia continued to attack during Catherine's reign. In the 1760s, this included Jean-Baptiste Chappe d'Auteroche, who traveled across Russia to Tobol'sk in Siberia in 1761 to observe the Transit of Venus. The first volume of Chappe d'Auteroche's account was a detailed description of his travel from France to Tobol'sk; the second volume was a series of short essays enumerating Russia's resources, including its minerals, geography, and peoples. Those essays were reliant on the available resources on Siberia, including Eberhard Isbrand Ides, Gmelin, and Strahlenberg. Steller's account of Kamchatka was published as the third volume of Chappe d'Auteroche's account but was left out of the English translation in 1770 because it had already been published there.[13] Relying on official Russian sources, particularly Ides and Gmelin, as proof of Russia's failure to manage its empire, revealed how dangerous the academy's work could be for the tsar's reputation.[14]

When Chappe d'Auteroche assessed "the population, trade, navy, revenues, and land forces of Russia," he began from a premise that most Enlightened thinkers would accept: "The power of the state arises from its population; altho' in many countries this circumstance is the least object of the attention of the government. Depravity of manners, luxury, and the wretchedness of the people, are the chief impediments to population; since it is well known, that unlawful connections contribute but little to the propagation of the species." Russia suffered from all these impediments, in addition to its well-known challenge: "In northern countries, the climate furnishes a fresh obstacle to population: the regions of the Laplanders, of the Samoiedes, and all the northern parts of Russia, have been always depopulated, and will ever be so, because of the unfruitfulness of the soil, and the bad quality of the food these people are obliged to live upon: this food contains hardly any nutritious juice, and all nature in these climates seems to be in a state of perpetual sluggishness, in which scarce any active principles are to be discovered" (figure 4.1). The extreme climate remained a perpetual obstacle. Chappe d'Auteroche also believed the climate reduced the procreative ability of its population, mentioning that "almost all philosophers are of opinion, that the constitution has less powerful influence in the northern, than in the southern climates: the people of the north are less addicted to venery."[15]

Echoing the observations of the earlier narratives, Chappe d'Auteroche believed that the Russians overcame the natural disinterest in sex among the people of the empire. He argued: "The Russians an exception to this general rule: and it should seem that this apparent contradiction may be accounted for from moral causes. The women being left to themselves, and suffered to live in idleness, the effects even of their most trifling passions must be powerful. Among the common people, men, women and

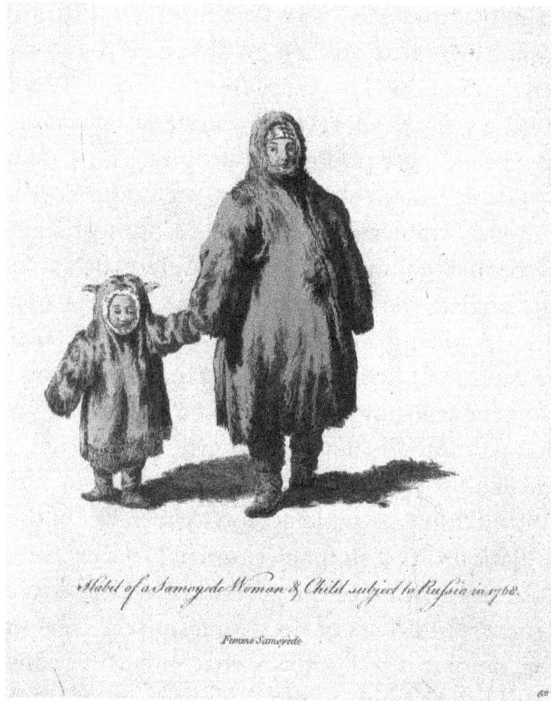

FIGURE 4.1. This illustration of a Samoyed woman and child was included in the French edition of Chappe d'Auteroche's text. In a section highlighting the Samoyed disinterest in procreation, including a child in the image highlighted the issue. "Habit of a Samoyede woman and child subject to Russia in 1768. Femme Samoyèd," The Miriam and Ira D. Wallach Division of Art, Prints and Photographs: Art and Architecture Collection, The New York Public Library, New York Public Library Digital Collections, accessed June 9, 2024, https://digitalcollections.nypl.org/items/510d47e4-7ef6-a3d9-e040-e00a18064a99.

children lie together promiscuously, without any sense of shame. Hence their passions being excited by the objects they see, the two sexes give themselves up early to debauchery." Chappe d'Auteroche was as interested in the sex lives of Russia's subjects as any of his predecessors, and he included innumerable details of the Russians' questionable morality throughout his travels. In Nizhnii Novgorod, for example, he mentioned "The young lads in this town, as well as in the neighbouring places, are married at fourteen or fifteen years of age, and the girls at thirteen: the women often breed 'till they are fifty." The reason for the young marriage age was not religious or cultural, but "necessary to marry the girls early, in order to prevent debauchery" (figure 4.2).[16]

If the Russians were marrying early, why was the population not larger? Chappe d'Auteroche argued that it was not because of the lack

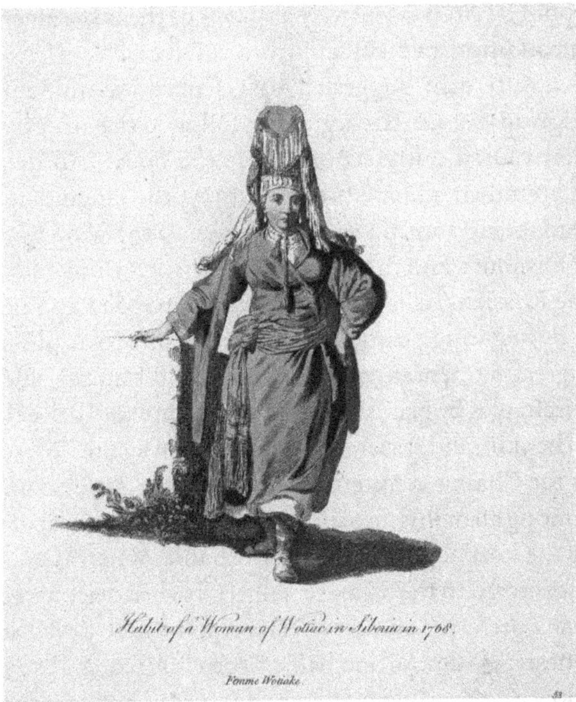

FIGURE 4.2. The previous Samoyed woman and child contrast with this Chuvash woman, one of the peoples of "northern Tartary" discussed in Chappe d'Auteroche's text (1757–1772). "Habit of a woman of Wotiac in Siberia in 1768. Femme Wotiake," The Miriam and Ira D. Wallach Division of Art, Prints and Photographs: Art and Architecture Collection, The New York Public Library, New York Public Library Digital Collections, accessed June 9, 2024, https://digitalcollections.nypl.org/items/42e2e440-c5fc-012f-f3f9-58d385a7bc34.

of sexual interest among the Siberian population, but rather the devastating effects of endemic diseases. Three were inescapable: smallpox, syphilis, and scurvy. Together, they "make so much havock in Russia, that unless the government takes some measures to prevent their effects, they will put an end to the human species in this country." His estimates on the outcome for the population were dire: "The small-pox carries off near one half of the children: this disease seems to have been communicated to this country from Europe"; in other words, Russians introduced and spread the disease across the country. "Venereal disorders are diffused throughout all Russia, and in northern Tartary more than any where else. The men are much addicted to sodomy in Russia. Venereal disorders prevail among all the people from St. Petersburg to Tobolsky." His evidence for the prevalence of syphilis came from

Gmelin, whom he cited extensively as proof of the government's awareness of the condition and its inability to resolve it[17]

Chappe d'Auteroche suggested that scurvy was undoubtedly the most widespread disease. His argument followed the accepted idea that cold weather caused putrefaction inside the body: "All the Russians, in general, are much addicted to the scurvy; the languid and inactive life they lead, being shut up in their stoves all the winter, make them very full of humours, and they perspire very little." Unlike smallpox and syphilis, the Russians' reliance on the bania provided a solution to the condition, by inspiring perspiration and releasing toxic humors. "They produce a great fermentation in the blood and humors, and bring on plentiful discharges by perspiration. The extreme cold drive the humors back from the skin, and restores the equilibrium again." What remained a question for Chappe d'Auteroche was why use of the bania had not extended among all of Russia's subjects, preferring the heat of their large stoves over the heat and humidity of the bania. Whereas every Russian "from the sovereign to the meanest subject, bathes twice a week," Tatars and Siberians preferred the stove. The results were devastating: "The small-pox destroys almost one half of the children, and some times a greater proportion" and syphilis was widespread and "more dangerous here than in any other place, on account of their being usually joined with the scurvy, and that the medicine proper for one of these diseases always increases the other." Without effective government intervention, these diseases "in the process of time should put an end to the human species in these parts."[18]

Chappe d'Auteroche included Ides's, Gmelin's, and Steller's texts as evidence; few, if any, of his observations were new. His conclusions, however, were. Building on more than a century of travel narratives and the more recent fieldwork by the academy, Chappe d'Auteroche presented a straightforward argument. Russia's inability to treat or prevent its endemic diseases not only led to an underpopulated empire but also threatened to exterminate the remaining population. Russia's failure to develop its natural resources was not a failure of science or engineering, but rather a public health crisis. Notably, other Frenchmen had made similar arguments about France's failures to control its disease burden at the same time, with the exact same consequences on the French populace.[19] If a difference was to be found in Chappe d'Auteroche's criticism, it might have been the timing of it—first critiquing the government for its ineffective rule and lack of concern for its population, and then the truth of Catherine's coup as proof of both problems. An anonymous refutation of Chappe d'Auteroche's text was published in Paris a year after its first edition in 1770, but no Russian official offered any public response.[20]

Privately, Catherine was not silent on the topic. Chappe d'Auteroche published his travel narrative in a period when Catherine was actively corresponding with other figures of the Enlightenment, including François-Marie Arouet, better known by his pen name Voltaire. Early in 1771, for example, Catherine wrote to Voltaire mentioning the great success she had in hosting the prince of Prussia in St. Petersburg, who admired the city's beauty, unlike "Abbé Chappe, who saw everything in Russia from a closed sledge, in which he travelled post-haste."[21] Catherine casually dismissed the idea of Chappe d'Auteroche's accuracy with her comment, suggesting he failed to see Siberia in any sense. Voltaire was a sympathetic audience. In a response to Catherine written later that same year, Voltaire mentioned he enjoyed the refutation of Chappe d'Auteroche's book that had been recently published. Furthermore, he praised the recent publication of Catherine's *Instruction* in a French translation, "which ought to belong to all the kings and tribunals in the world." The *Instruction* had been censored in Paris by "some ill-mannered cur," but, for Voltaire, that was only further evidence of Russia's superiority to France.[22]

Nothing stated by Catherine's French critics was markedly different from the ongoing private conversations throughout her court. The British diplomats, in particular, were strikingly critical of the Russian political system, but Britain, unlike France, remained dependent on Russia's exports, leaving these indictments as private advice provided to the foreign secretary by the ambassadors.[23] George Macartney served in St. Petersburg in the early years of Catherine's reign and described Catherine's court as filled "with the most provoking Phlegm & the most Stoical Indifference."[24] In other words, the people were phlegmatic and melancholic, and therefore disinterested in his negotiations. He continued by suggesting to the British foreign secretary that "you may imagine the Law of Nations can't have made any great Progress in a Country where there are no such thing as a University. Barbarous as they are & ignorant of those Arts which improve the understanding, enlighten the mind or promote discovery. . . . Like Children they are allured by every new Idea—pursue it for a moment & then abandon it when another starts up in their Imaginations."[25] Pointing toward Russian ignorance and immaturity only supported Chappe d'Auteroche's publication, but this description was offered by Russia's closest European ally.

Macartney's successor, Henry Shirley, was hardly any kinder. In a dispatch to the foreign secretary sent in 1768, he reported on Catherine's Legislative Assembly, currently meeting in Moscow to discuss potential reforms. It was an explicit indictment: "The manner in which they have hitherto proceeded in attempting so many important affairs & so very difficult, appeared to me so much like a Farce, that it would have been ridiculous to fill up several Sheets with an Account of Things which can only pique, & not interest Our Curiosity, raised by the noisy Flatterers of thos Men who are struck by mere appearances, or who scrape some advantages by offering up Incense to this Idol of the Empress's Vanity."[26] After outlining the combined disaster of Catherine's lack of leadership and the assembly's inability to solve Russia's challenges, Shirley could only offer his regrets: "One cannot help pitying the Russians, who think themselves so wise, so powerful, when they are such an immense Distance from the happy situations of some Nations of Europe."[27] Although Shirley did not explicitly connect the cold climate to the political shortcomings, his assessment of Russia still agreed with Montesquieu's view.

Russia's critics argued that the cold climate was an unavoidable challenge for the bodies and intellect of the empire. It was responsible for the procreative challenge that resulted in an underpopulated state. It facilitated the spread of three endemic diseases that further reduced the population. It is arguable, at least, that following the Second Kamchatka Expedition, the academy, if not the government itself, took steps to finding effective therapies to mitigate, or even cure, both scurvy and syphilis. Even at the time, the results of those treatments were debatable, but the government could make an argument it was aware and working to address two of Chappe d'Auteroche's problems. By the time of his travel across Russia in 1762, however, the other two (smallpox and the low birth rate) were not yet the focus of the academy or the state's attentions. If the Russian Empire was going to improve its health and increase its population, those issues needed to be addressed as soon as possible.

Public Interventions

The Russian Empire was not waiting for foreign critics before intervening to improve the health of the population. Early travelers, and the academy's expedition, had already been investigating conditions inside the empire and recommending actions. The Russian government may have preferred physicians trained in certain schools, but neither the staff nor the curriculum at those schools was stagnant. Medical knowledge was constantly evolving. The first major reform of Russia's education system arrived after Nicolaas Bidloo's death, with the new curriculum designed by Dr. Johann Bernhard Fischer on December 24, 1735. Fischer was born in Lubeck in 1685 and would pursue medicine at Halle, Jena, and Leiden, where he studied with Herman Boerhaave and completed his medical doctorate with a thesis, "About Mania," in 1705. In 1710, Fischer established a practice in Riga, and was brought into Russia through Peter the Great's conquest of that city. Under Russian rule he prospered, becoming Anna Ivanovna's personal physician in 1735. His reform plan for hospitals was a lengthy document that outlined in detail the responsibilities of each rank of employee as well as the responsibilities of its students. The hospitals would be led by a physician and supported by a head surgeon, five surgeons, ten recent graduates, and twenty surgical students as well as one apothecary.[28] The responsibilities of each rank of employee was listed to clarify the relationship between these men and their patients.

Although the treatment of patients was not the primary purpose of this reform, Fischer notably included a table describing the ideal patient's diet while under treatment in the hospital. Bread, meat, and salt were prescribed every day, as well as one mug of beer and one glass of wine. Three times a week, the patients would be served oats, barley would be served once, and butter would be served four times.[29] In the eighteenth century, wine was utilized as a safe substance as a base ingredient for pharmaceutical preparations, but the rest reflected an ideal diet more than a specific therapeutic treatment. Later, as the director of the Medical Chancellery, Fischer authored a few books on medical treatments distributed to army surgeons. Between the reform of the hospital schools and his instruction manuals, his advice had a long legacy on Russian medical practice.

Twenty-five years after Fischer's reform, the medical curriculum would be updated again. The first change came from Elizaveta Petrovna's (r. 1741–1762) personal physician, Jean Armand de L'Estocq. Born and educated in Germany, and descended from a French noble family, L'Estocq arrived in Russia in 1709, becoming one of Peter the Great's court physicians and a confident of Elizaveta during Peter's reign.[30] L'Estocq was sent into internal exile during Anna Ivanovna's reign, but he returned following Elizaveta's seizure of the throne in 1741.[31] As *archiater*, or the head of the College of Medicine under

Elizaveta, L'Estocq added a new course in obstetrics as part of the Russian medical curriculum taught at the surgical schools established in Moscow and St. Petersburg in the 1750s.[32] This reform preceded the criticism of Russia's birth rate by Chappe d'Auteroche, but certainly this issue had been raised by the fieldwork conducted during the Second Kamchatka Expedition. At first glance, adding obstetrics to the medical curriculum only in the 1750s might have appeared to be a late development, but this was roughly concurrent with its addition to the medical curriculum at the University of Edinburgh, where several other Russian physicians, including L'Estocq's colleague John Cook, were trained. The curricular addition was supported by the state hiring its first two gynecologists, Gotthard Wilhem Reichardt and Andreas Lindemann, in 1757. Both men were born in the Russian Empire, Reichardt in Riga and Lindemann in Reval, but they received their medical degrees in Germany.[33]

The addition of obstetrics was not the end of the changes of that decade. L'Estocq's successor as archiater, James Mounsey, passed further revisions. Mounsey studied medicine at the University of Edinburgh, but did not graduate, instead becoming an apprentice to a local surgeon, Thomas Wood. In 1736, he entered Russian service, first working in the St. Petersburg Admiralty Hospital and then serving in the army in Ukraine. He would then receive his medical doctorate at the University of Reims, France, before returning to Russia in 1741, where he returned to army service. By 1756, he was sufficiently well known among Russia's elite to be sent by Elizaveta Petrovna to care for Ernst Johann Biron's wife. Following the death of Elizaveta's court physician, Mounsey became the new court physician and a state councilor in 1760. Following Elizaveta's death the following year, Tsar Peter III promoted Mounsey to archiater.[34]

Shortly after his new appointment, Mounsey issued two significant changes to the operations of the medical establishment. The first was a set of guidelines to recognize medical service in parallel with the existing Table of Ranks, so that medical practitioners could advance through the social system following similar guides for the army or navy, which was approved by the Senate in February 1762. The second was an "Instruction to All Doctors on the Discharge of Their Duties," which was signed by Peter III and approved by the College of Medicine on April 30, 1762. This instruction added an incentive for doctors that could "describe, draw and collect animal vegetable or mineral specimens of natural history or *materia medica*, particularly in remote areas."[35] In other words, it was a formal directive to continue the work begun by Daniel Gottlieb Messerschmidt, Gmelin, and Steller. Unfortunately for Mounsey, when Catherine overthrew her husband, she also removed Mounsey from the Medical College in her general dismissal of all of Peter's ministers, even if the official reason was Mounsey's "ill health."[36]

During his time in Russia, Mounsey was an active correspondent, publishing several notes in the Royal Society's *Philosophical Transactions* and submitting suggestions to the new Royal Society for Arts, Manufactures, and Commerce.[37] In Britain, his contributions to natural history, both from his involvement in exporting rhubarb from Russia and attempted investigation of the source of castor, were known.[38] In terms of his Russian career, however, his medical expertise may have been more significant. In 1748, for example, he published case notes on the treatment of a woman "from Whom a Foetus Was Extracted." It involved an unnamed "Soldier's Wife" in Finland in 1742. Her symptoms began in September 1741, when "she felt a Pain beneath the Navel, with a Swelling and Redness, which in about three Weeks appear'd like a small Boil. This she pierced with an Awl, and a yellow-colour'd Water ran from it without any Smell, and continued so to do for near three Weeks more, when it discharged a purulent stinking Matter." The following June, eight months after these initial symptoms, "two small Bones came out, which were given to the Surgeon that visited her; who only applied a Piece of Plaister, persuading her that a Cure was impossible."[39]

In October 1742, "this unhappy Woman applied to Dr. Mounsey, who, after a careful Examination, undertook to deliver her." The initial surgery that followed was unsuccessful, because "she being unruly, and the Operation not going on to the Doctor's Liking," the procedure was halted, "only some loose Bones were extracted." The following day, the Army surgeon and Mounsey continued, with a larger incision making "a large Opening" from which a "fetus" was extracted, comprised of "matter" that "had a very nauseous Smell, and continued of Membranes, Fat, and corrupted Flesh." At that point, the operation "having been long, and the Woman fainting away, the Wound was dressed, without attempting to extract more at that time. In the Evening she was taken with Vomitings; but by proper internal Medicines, and Flannel Stoups were wrung out of hot Wine, applied over the whole Belly, and often renew'd, she found Ease, and grew better." The next day, a third surgery followed, removing "the Bones of the Trunk, and most of the other large ones, with their Ligaments and rotten Flesh, were taken out. The Matter discharged for several Days was of a dark-brown Colour, occasion'd by Blood issuing from the dilated Pores of the internal Surface of the Sack." Mounsey's conclusion was that the "sack" was one of the fallopian tubes. Remarkably, the "Wound was cured in about six Weeks, and the Woman deliver'd from a long State of Misery grew fat and lusty, and now enjoys good Health."[40]

There was no question to Mounsey that the woman's earlier illness, in September 1741, was directly linked to the surgeries that followed in October 1742. The idea of this woman surviving an ectopic pregnancy for thirteenth months seemed plausible to him. Equally remarkable, "the Woman came by Sea to Stockholm above a Year after this Cure [the three surgeries], and was presented to the Academy in good Health; and the Doctor [Mounsey] believes she is still alive and well."[41] As evidence of the accuracy of this account, Mounsey and Sir George Baker included a citation to the original publication of the incident in the *Acts* of the Swedish Royal Academy, which was the location of the final examination of this astonishing patient.

Very little of this case study could be truthful according to modern medicine. Surviving an ectopic pregnancy for four months would be remarkable now, much less then. Surviving three surgical procedures in short succession, without anesthesia, in the 1740s would be implausible, if not impossible. Because Mounsey was involved in the case, it seems reasonable to assume the details he observed were accurate, but he was not involved in the surgeries, just the diagnosis and recovery, nor was he involved in the original examination the previous year. It is likely this case is a collection of disconnected incidents, or even manufactured ones. Considering the timing of this publication in connection with addition of obstetrics to the Russian medical curriculum in the 1750s, however, reveals more about the medical establishment's intentions than it does about the accuracy of the details. The Russian Academy not only was focusing on a curricular change but also had employed leading specialists in the field. Mounsey's rise through the ranks to become head of the College of Medicine confirmed this commitment.

Catherine's dismissal of Mounsey did not change the pace of medical reform. Her government turned to a different British man, Daniel Dumaresq, the former chaplain of the Russia Company in St. Petersburg, to supervise the design and implementation of the new curriculum in 1765.[42] Dumaresq had been involved with Catherine's son's education, and he had gained some attention for his scientific work by publishing a summary of Stepan Krasheninnikov's findings on the Kamchatka Expedition in *Philosophical Transactions* in 1759.[43]

Catherine and Dumaresq's medical education reform was followed by new guidelines on best practices for childbirth in 1766, maintaining the state's commitment to improving the birth rate.[44] Two years later, further changes were promulgated for the medical curriculum at the hospital schools. The government required the College of Medicine to hire translators to support importing more medical treatises from Europe. It also confirmed the continuing importance of maintaining the anatomy theaters and botanical gardens attached to the hospital schools, leaving the preexisting curriculum intact.[45] These changes led to a dramatic transformation of Russia's medical knowledge. In the historian S. M. Grombakh's study of Russia's medical literature in the eighteenth century, he uncovered only seven printed medical texts in Russian before 1760s. Thirty-four texts were published in the next decade alone, and this number would only increase for the remainder of the century.[46] Foreign specialists had always been part of Russia's medical establishment at the state level, but Catherine's government focused on disseminating their knowledge to Russia's medical corps in Russian, theoretically making this material more accessible than ever before.

Montesquieu critiqued Russia's government as a by-product of a cold climate, and Chappe d'Auteroche followed with a scathing indictment of Russia's manifold failures as an imperial power in Siberia. Both men wrote, however, during a period when the Russian government was invested in improving its public health. More of a surprise may be the equally critical assessments by the British, despite the prominent role British physicians occupied in Russia, including several archiaters of the College of Medicine. After Mounsey was removed from office, he was no less judgmental than his fellow diplomats had been: "The State of Learning in this country is scarce yet out of the cradle however knowledge is become justly universal but it is mostly Superficial. There have been many things translated into Russ within these few years But authors in the original Russ are none considerable besides some pieces of Poetry which are said to be very good. The Genius of the Nation is quick and apt to learn, But they make more progress in the Beaux Arts than in Abstract Learning, and it will be many years before they make any figure that near."[47] The Academy of Sciences sponsored expeditions that searched for methods to mitigate the damage of scurvy and syphilis; new specialists were hired and the medical curriculum was updated to improve the birth rate of the empire. Public health had become an imperial concern, even if Russia's critics had not noticed.

Solving Smallpox

Smallpox was the major pandemic of the eighteenth century. Mortality rates globally reached new highs. Historians of disease have speculated that it was during the century that the primary variant of smallpox circulating globally became *variola major* rather than *variola minor*, as a way to explain the mortality spike, but this theory remains unproven. Before the eighteenth century, inoculating against smallpox may have been unknown in Europe, but several methods had been adopted globally. News of a potential inoculation method reached Britain in 1714, when Emanuel Timonius, an Italian-educated physician in practice in Constantinople, reported his knowledge to a college in the Royal Society of London; this method was published in English in *Philosophical Transactions* shortly thereafter. According to Timonius, "The Circassians, Georgians, and other Asiaticks, have introduc'd this practice of procuring the Small-Pox by a sort of Inoculation." His recommendation was to find a "some Boy, or young Lad, of a sound healthy Temperament, that is seized with the common Small-Pox," then "press out the Matter coming from them," and then inject that pus into "several little Wounds with a Needle."[48] Following further endorsements from other physicians, a domestic trial was begun and shortly thereafter the royal family would be inoculated. The general public in Britain, however, did not immediately seek the treatment, though domestic clinics continued to operate.[49]

Skeptics of the procedure had some justification. In theory, patients were to be inoculated with the pox from a mild case (or "common" to Timonius). In the eighteenth century, it was left to the doctor's discretion to identify mild symptoms. Now, we might classify these types as *variola major* and *variola minor*, but the two forms had not been identified yet. Because *major* had a mortality rate of 30 percent and *minor* a mortality rate of only 1 percent, the risks for using *variola major* were significant. Furthermore, the pox used for the variolation procedure needed to be live rather than dried, and so a patient with active pox needed to be used as the source for treatment. The solution for gathering viable pox was to identify patients in the midst of an ongoing smallpox outbreak, harvest the pox, and inoculate their uninfected neighbors, because the pox could not be stored for future use. The long-term solution was to infect, intentionally, patients to have a ready supply on hand. The solution for an ample supply of previously uninfected patients adopted by British practitioners was to infect orphans in pairs in case one died from the procedure. An orphan's inability to object to being the subject of a dangerous medical treatment made them appealing incubators for the medical establishment.[50]

Even after reaching the highest level of Europe's nobility, other elites continued to resist inoculation. This resistance occurred despite the clear and present danger of a smallpox outbreak. Tsar Peter II of Russia died from the disease on his wedding day at the age of fourteen in 1730, leading to the succession crisis that would bring Anna Ivanovna to the throne. The British consul's wife, Jane Ward, suggested Peter's infection began with an unfortunate cold: "As soon as they got into the room, the emperor complained of the head-ach; this was at first taken to proceed from the cold, but on repeated complaints, his physician was called; . . . The next day the small pox appeared on the emperor, and on the nineteenth, the day appointed for his marriage, about three in the morning, he died."[51] Even in Britain, however, inoculation to prevent smallpox made progress with the broader public only in the 1740s, too late for young Peter II.[52]

By the middle of the century, a British physician, Daniel Sutton, had developed a new method of variolating that he believed was less risky than the initial version that had been practiced.[53] Sutton's method involved extensive preparation of the patients and up to two weeks of treatment after inoculation. It began with a "Preparative Powder" composed of calomel (mercury chloride), magnesium carbonate, and cinnabar (mercury sulfite) administered in the evening, followed by salts and water to induce stools the following morning. After five days of this treatment, the patient was prepared for inoculation. As he described the procedure, "hold the launcet, with the flat side upwards, between your forefinger and thumb, just moisten the tip with the [variolous] matter, and then make two small punctures in the arm, about two inches a part, wipe the launcet on the punctures, and it is done; if the blood starts the puncture is deep enough." Following the procedure, patients were given a "Repellent Pill," made of Kermes minerals (a mixture of antimony trioxide and antimony trisulfide), powdered Aloe succotrina, and camphire (henna), mixed with wine. On alternating nights until the rash and symptoms had passed completely, the patient would also take "grey powder," which was the mercury-based preparative powder without cinnabar. Sutton's emphasis in his directions was that the proper powders needed to be administered, but recovery would be supported if the patients were not allowed any butter or meat until "the twelfth or thirteenth day after Inoculation," but only could have "toast and water" before that date. He also was concerned that patients should not be allowed to "sit hot by the fire especially during their Sickening, for it will increase both their symptoms and the number of Pustules." In fact, "Every Person should walk out in the air often every day"; and, if necessary, they should be taken outside even if "they let their Heads be ever so bad."[54] Sutton's adjusted his treatment to be able to inoculate children as young as six months, and accounted for differences in "strong" and "delicate" constitutions, making it potentially viable for everyone.

Within only a few years, other British physicians began simplifying Sutton's method, primarily cutting costs by reducing the number of expensive medicines. In 1766, Sir George Baker, then the royal physician, described the Suttonian Method of variolation only requiring cold, fresh air. According to Baker, neither the expensive chemical preparations nor the adjustment to the diet was necessary, and he found no evidence of a distinction between an incision and a puncture.[55] The following year, Dr. Thomas Dimsdale published *The Present Method for Inoculating the Small-Pox*, presenting himself as the expert of this new method, advocating for Sutton's procedure but also reducing its cost, though not as radically as Baker. Drug preparations would be given less frequently, and young children and those with delicate constitutions should not be inoculated.[56] By removing those most likely to suffer from the procedure, Dimsdale's revised method produced fewer deaths than Sutton's original clinic.

Considering the historical ties between Russia and Britain, and between the Academy of Sciences and the Royal Society of London, the Russian Empire had multiple opportunities to understand the benefits of variolation as a therapy and a public campaign to inoculate the population. The Second Kamchatka Expedition observed smallpox across the empire, including its devasting consequences for the Indigenous populations of Siberia and Kamchatka. Those consequences were exploited by Chappe d'Auteroche in his condemnation of Russian imperial practices. In 1762 when Chappe d'Auteroche traveled to Tobol'sk, the Russian government had yet to adopt a solution to the smallpox pandemic; by the time he published his critique in 1768, however, Catherine the Great's government had embarked on an ambitious plan to inoculate the public. Meanwhile, the Parlement of Paris had banned inoculation in 1763. It was in fact the French government, rather than Russia's government, that was risking the public's health with its inaction.[57]

With all the changes to medical practice that had begun in the 1750s and continued during the early years of Catherine's reign in the 1760s, the decision to adopt public inoculation against smallpox should not be a surprise.[58] There was both a lengthy history of the danger of the disease in Russia as well as an immediate threat to the court. Countess Anna Petrovna Sheremeteva, Count Panin's fiancé, fell "very dangerously ill" just before their wedding in 1768. Panin was forced to depart from the house they shared for fear of potentially exposing Catherine.[59] Sheremeteva died within two weeks of her diagnosis. The British ambassador would describe her as "a young Lady of uncommon merit, beautiful, and immensely rich."[60] Catherine had personally intervened to arrange for Sheremeteva's divorce from her first husband to allow her marriage to Panin. Dimsdale would later confirm that Sheremeteva's death and Catherine's potential exposure inspired Catherine's decision to hire an inoculator that year. As Dimsdale detailed, once it was known that "neither rank nor fortune afforded any security against the ravages of this dreadful disease; and the whole court, sensible of the danger to which the Empress and the Grand Duke were exposed, were filled with extreme solicitude for those lives upon which the safety and happiness of the empire so essentially depended."[61]

The Russian government did not consider hiring the inventor of the new method, Sutton, but rather the English physician who promoted himself as the expert in the procedure, Dimsdale. Dimsdale was not Scottish as had been the overwhelming majority of British physicians at work Russia, nor was he born or educated in Germany as was the majority of the medical establishment. His hiring broke all the established networks that had placed specialists in Russia. It is likely that his publishing record, rather than his connections to men already working in Russia, was the key. We must consider the possibility that part of the appeal of Dimsdale in Russia was an expectation that he would publicize the government's commitment to variolation. Given that Dismdale published a series of tracts explaining his success in Russian in St. Petersburg and in English in London, he did exactly that. Dimsdale's recorded successes, however, were based on avoiding general inoculation to treat only the few who were the most likely to recover quickly. Dimsdale's impact on the health of the general public may have been nominal at the time but was significant for the health of the court.

According to Dimsdale's later account, Catherine desired a specialist trained in the Suttonian Method to inoculate herself and the royal family. Dimsdale was proud that the Russian ambassador to Britain,

Aleksei Semenovich Musin-Pushkin, came to hire him personally at his clinic in Britain in 1768. If Catherine did desire a Suttonian specialist, few options were available, as the therapy was brand new and not widely used outside of Sutton's clinic at the time. Dimsdale's narrative presented his choice to enter Russian service as an opportunity to benefit humanity, and not for "lucrative motives," but rather he acted "entirely to the gracious pleasure of her Imperial Majesty." He departed on July 28, 1768, taking his son, who was currently in medical school in Edinburgh, to act as his assistant.[62]

In Dimsdale's recollection of his time in Russia, he acted professionally and quickly to prepare Catherine and her court for the treatment. Dimsdale suggested first "inoculating some of her [Catherine's] own sex, and age, and as near as could be of similar habit" to observe the consequences of inoculation in a different climate than England's, but "the Empress replied, 'that if the practice had been novel, or the least doubt of the general success had remained, that precaution might be necessary'; but as she was well satisfied in both particulars, there would be no occasion for delay on any account."[63] Despite Catherine's confidence, Dimsdale was more cautious in the application of his methods and set up a short clinical trial to adjust to the new conditions.

The trial was held at the house of the former head of the Russia Company, Baron Wolff, transformed into Russia's first smallpox clinic, which Catherine purchased for this purpose.[64] "Dr. Schulenius, a physician of Livonia, who had successfully inoculated many persons in that province, in a method similar to that which was formerly practiced in England, was engaged to live there, and superintend the patients; as also Dr. Strenge to act as his colleague in that employment."[65] According to a later account, Schulenius began inoculating in Dorpat "in the year 1756, and practised it with so much success in the country round him, that within eight years he had inoculated 1023 children, of whom only one died."[66] Despite Schulenius's experience and successes, the new clinic implemented the Suttonian Method with punctures rather than incisions. Schulenius was left to run the clinic, while Dimsdale stayed at the court. Dimsdale's son, only a medical student, remained at the clinic to supervise the procedures and update his father on its progress. The staff began inoculating with

> two young gentlemen of the cadet's corps, . . . whose names were Basoff and Swieten, about the age of fourteen years (who were supposed not to have had the small pox) were accordingly inoculated.

> I say supposed, because, however strange it may appear, at that time the nature and symptoms of the disease were so little known and attended to, there were few who could be certain whether they ever had had this disease or not. The general method was to search for marks, and if none were found, it was concluded the party had not had the disease.

Both cadets recovered from the disease within a week, which led Dimsdale to conclude the first experiment was perfect. Consent, however, was not a concern of the physicians. These two cadets were assigned to the inoculation by the court. Dimsdale was later surprised to discover that, in recovery, the cadets "considered themselves as victims devoted to a dangerous experiment," which Dimsdale blamed on a fever "which might probably increase the patient's apprehensions."[67]

Dimsdale's subsequent actions, however, confirm that his focus was on preparing Catherine and her court for a safe inoculation, not on the general well-being of his other patients. The two cadets were followed by four more, "and a young maid servant of our family," who also lacked the opportunity to object to the treatment. All were chosen "as proper subjects for inoculation, and the natural small-pox, in a suitable state for the purpose, was discovered in the suburbs of the city." In the suburbs, a court surgeon had found a small child, who "was rather full of small-pox; the kind was favourable and distinct, and near the time of maturation," but he was being kept in a house that was too hot, leaving him "gasping for breath." To Dimsdale, this was proof of Russia's "improper manner of treating the disease, and the prejudices of the populace," as the Suttonian Method required patients to be kept in a space with cool air and good ventilation.[68]

The heat, however, was not Dimsdale's only objection to this treatment. When Dimsdale approached the child with a needle "to take the matter for inoculation, a woman, whom I was soon informed was the mother of child, threw herself on her knees at my feet, with her forehead on the ground, and her arms over her head (the eastern manner of prostration, which is still retained in Russia) in this posture she made a plaintive cry, in a language I did not understand." The woman, apparently, was under the impression gathering material for inoculation would lead to the death of her son. Although Dimsdale was "shocked at the thought of being considered a murderer," he informed the surgeon to assure the woman that no harm would come to her son, and then he proceeded to inoculate all of five of his subjects.[69]

Dimsdale's second experiment was not a success. The five patients all "appeared to be infected by the operation," but none developed the illness after a week.[70] His hypothesis was that all must have been exposed to smallpox earlier in their lives, but unfortunately had failed to show any telltale marks to demonstrate their previous infection. As he later complained to the British ambassador, his "first patients had so little eruption that tho' he was convinced many of them really had the small pox, it was difficult to propagate the Distemper from them."[71] Dimsdale rejected an argument that suggested Russians constant use of the bathhouse led to "increased flow of perspiration" that might have provided some protection.[72] The Suttonian Method relied on cold, fresh air, rather than heat, making the bania particularly suspect. To prove his theory, Dimsdale ordered his staff to inoculate each of the five subjects a second time, "in the old and original manner, still practised by Dr. Schulenius, by a long incision, in which lint moistened with matter was inserted, and the wound covered with a plaister. I recommended likewise, that the patients should frequent the rooms of those who were under the natural small-pox, even of the worst sort; that they should touch the sick, and use every means that might expose them to receive the disease."[73] Dimsdale's disregard for his patients' health is not surprising in an eighteenth-century context. Neither the cadets, who belonged to state service, nor his own maid could have opted out of the treatment. Dimsdale's only concern was Catherine and her court; he took the necessary steps to treat his royal patron, not her subjects.

Despite the failure of Dimsdale's second trial, Catherine instructed him to move forward with her treatment. Therefore, he "selected and inoculated three children of good constitutions, to be ready, as near as could be computed, at the time agreed on." These subjects were cared for in the makeshift hospital, and when the infection reached the proper stage, one of the children was taken while asleep to the palace, where "the inoculation was soon performed, after which my son returned back to Wolf House, with the child, and intimated to the family there (who were anxious to know what had been done), that I had inoculated the child of a nobleman."[74] It was perhaps not necessary for the child's parents to know that she had been used to inoculate Catherine the Great, but it is notable that they also were not informed when their daughter was taken from the hospital. Dimsdale's inoculation was a medical success but was facilitated by a kidnapping. Although Dimsdale was "sworn to secrecy" about Catherine's procedure, regular updates circulated around the court.[75] Following her treatment, Catherine "who has only had the slightest Indisposition, and has never been confined to Her Apartment since the Operation, had . . . a very favorable Eruption of the small Pox, very few in Number, and of a Quality entirely to Doctor Dimsdales Satisfaction."[76]

From a modern perspective, his methods are questionable at best, if not criminal, but without doubt that Catherine the Great considered her inoculation a success. Once she recovered, she described her decision to be inoculated in a letter to Voltaire, having "thought the best thing for to do would be for [her] to set a personal example which might be of use to people." Following Dimsdale's procedure, she did "not have a moment's illness, and have been receiving people every day." Confidently she proclaimed, "everyone wants to be inoculated; a bishop is going to have it done, and more people have been inoculated here in one month than in eight at Vienna."[77] Voltaire had been a long-term advocate for inoculation, having included an essay on the topic in his *Letters concerning the English Nation* (1733).[78] Catherine could hardly have chosen a better audience for her first report on the success of her procedure.

More information was made publicly available in Russia the following year. Surprisingly, the first printed text in Russian on inoculation was a description of the "German" method that had been set aside by Dimsdale's new version.[79] This first text, however, was shortly followed by an official publication by the Senate that detailed Dimsdale's "brief and clear instructions" on his new method of extracting pus from live pox and injecting the material into the arm as the correct method.[80] By the end of 1770, only two years after Catherine's treatment, two more pamphlets written by Dimsdale and translated into Russian were published by the Academy of Sciences, leaving little debate about which method of inoculation would be deployed across the empire.[81]

Considering the sheer size of the Russian Empire, it could not be a quick achievement to inoculate the population. Dimsdale was a strong advocate for expanding the inoculation program across the empire as soon as possible, but he expected the government to intervene in each village individually, without considering the logistics of that plan. Although he was confident noble families would easily undertake their inoculations at home, "the poor cannot enjoy those advantages. Humanity, however, and the interest of the state equally demand, that all possible attention should be bestowed for their assistance and preservation." Dimsdale recommended the Russian Empire follow a "certain method" he had employed in Britain. The government should prepare a list of every person in each village, by name, sex, and age, and mark whether or not they had recovered from smallpox previously. With that list, one physician could enter the village, variolate everyone who had yet to be exposed "on the same day: and, if this be performed in a proper manner, they might be all duly visited, and proper medicines administered at a moderate expence, and the whole be over in about three weeks: after which, that village would have nothing to apprehend from the small-pox soon after its birth, or that inoculation should be performed in every town or village once in five or six years."[82]

It was not that his plan was not sensible, but it required information the Russian government simply did not collect on a systematic basis. The first general census of the Russian Empire would not occur until the end of the nineteenth century. Multiple district or regional tax assessments could have included demographic data as early as the seventeenth century, but that process would have needed to be overhauled to gather the correct information, keep it up to date, and effectively centralize and collate the data. Then a sufficient number of medical practitioners would need to be employed to cover Russia's vast expanse, and, somehow, the new administrative staff, medical practitioners, and necessary supplies would need to be financed. If that was not challenge enough, smallpox would need to be kept live to allow variolation. Was Dimsdale's plan to forcibly seize more children? Would they take serfs? Recruits from the army? None of these necessary decisions were included in his plan. To be fair, no country in the world had managed this type of system on a national scale by the 1770s. It may be inspiring that Dimsdale assumed Russia could be the first.

The state persisted in the expansion of inoculation across Russia in the 1770s, but hardly on the scale Dimsdale expected. A journal published a discussion of the inoculation process in 1772, disseminating knowledge to the literate public, to support the expansion of the treatment.[83] The first clinic outside of St. Petersburg was established in Moscow, where one of its hospitals established a specialized wing for inoculating children. English minister and traveler William Coxe visited the city in the fall of 1778 and was impressed that the public hospital in the city had a facility "capable of containing 200 children" during treatment.[84] Samuel Bentham, an Englishman hired to inspect the mines in Siberia by the College of Manufacturing, observed physicians inoculating the Indigenous populations of Siberia during his tour of the region in 1781. When he traveled to Kiakhta on the Chinese border, he noted a physician from Irkutsk inoculating the community of Tatars near Bratsk, demonstrating that the instruction issued in the previous decade was still being following.[85] By the time that Catherine's government issued its general directive for the inoculation of the public in October 1787, which was upheld and reissued by the Senate the following spring, a significant, empirewide investment had been made in making the procedure available to the general public, not only for the Russians but also for the other imperial populations.[86] This is not intended to provide an overly optimistic view of smallpox treatment in Russia. While St. Petersburg, Moscow, Kyiv, Kazan', and Irkutsk had inoculation clinics established, the scale of the empire left considerable space between these treatment centers.[87]

The establishment of these few clinics across the empire was still a notable achievement, as Russia acted in advance of most European nations in terms of its commitment to smallpox inoculation. Russia's success was a surprise, even to its court. As the British ambassador wrote, "The ancient Russ has a great Dislike to Inoculation, as Mr. Panin espoused it, the Question might have become serious, had not the firmness and address of the Empress and her Minister got the better of all opposition."[88] Catherine's commitment to the process, however, did not mean that everyone shared its confidence in the process. Variolation, after all, was still a controversial treatment.

Given the remarkable freedom Dimsdale was given to run his smallpox trials, establish variolation clinics, and seize children from their homes to produce the pox, it might be expected that the value of inoculation was well understood. The devastation done by the disease in the Russian Empire had been a key topic for decades, raised by both Russia's specialists and foreign critics. Dimsdale, although hired to guide the solution, acknowledged that it was "impossible for me to ascertain with any degree of certainty, the precise number of persons who die annually of the small-pox in Russia." He instead projected a mortality rate from his knowledge of London's rate, "which enjoyed many advantages" that Russia lacked; therefore, Russia's rate must be worse. His prediction that "two million souls" died from smallpox each year in Russia seems impossibly high. His concern, however, was not the total loss of life, but rather "how much riches and strength of states depend upon the number of inhabitants. But perhaps there is not any country in which the certainty of this position is more indisputable than in Russia; for not only the strength of the empire, but the riches of every individual also, must be in proportion to the degree of population." Therefore, any loss of life from smallpox "must greatly retard the increase of the human species."[89]

After successfully treating the court, Catherine rewarded Dimsdale with the title of baron the following year, given "in justice to the rare Merit and skill of Thomas Dimsdale English gentleman & Doctor of Physic, whose humanity, Virtue & laudable Concern for the good of mankind in General, induced him long since to apply all his Thoughts, & Faculties towards improving and perfecting the Inoculation of the small Pox as they only Rational Preservation of the human Species from the destructive consequences of that mortal Disease."[90] According to the patent of his baronage, Dimsdale not only inoculated the court but also "destroy'd at the same time that baleful Hydra Prejudice & the dreadful apprehensions of this hitherto Fatal Disease." In recognition of his accomplishments, Catherine the Great's government awarded him with a new title, the rank of counsellor of state, and a pension for life of five hundred pounds per year.[91] Smallpox inoculation was personally profitable for Dimsdale.

In his published *Tracts on Inoculation*, Dimsdale argued that all attempts to preserve human life had value because the people were the wealth of the state. It was not an argument he made alone, as it was a recurring idea of the Enlightened era. French critics attacked Russia for its extreme climate and its propensity for autocracy and for its responsibility for introducing venereal disease and smallpox to Siberia and the North Pacific, where they threatened to eliminate the population. The Russian government, however, was making steady progress addressing its health woes following the evidence gathered on the Second Kamchatka Expedition. More scientific and medical information was imported, the medical curriculum was reformed, and new specialists were hired. By the 1750s if not earlier, the state had committed to increasing the population. Dimsdale's very public career was the cap on two decades of progress, not an uncertain first step.

Part III

Challenging Knowledge

CHAPTER 5

Surviving Plague, Mixing Races

In the spring of 1771, Russia was both figuratively and literally burning. It was at war with the Ottoman Empire while also threatening to invade Poland. The war exposed the Russian army to the bubonic plague, just as it had in 1710 and 1737. This new outbreak, however, was much worse, reaching as far north as Moscow, despite Russia's implementation of a quarantine along the border. At the same time, a series of fires burned in St. Petersburg in which arson was suspected. The British ambassador mentioned the first of the fires on May 24, when "a very great number of Wooden Houses and some Brick ones have been burnt; The Hotel of the Corps of the Marine Cadets are of the number and also a Hemp Warehouse." The ambassador was informed that fires "frequently happen at this season when there is no rain, the Wood of the Houses having been much heated by the Stoves in Winter, and therefore having great Power."[1] Three days later the situation was more ominous. There had been "successive Fires every Day . . . both in the Town and adjacent Villages, many of which are entirely consumed. It has been suspected that these fires are not accidental."[2] With the arrival of the plague, the ongoing military conflicts, and the calamitous fires, any government would struggle to respond. The ambassador prioritized the immediate risk of arson, but the other issues were far more pressing, both for Russians living in Moscow and Ukrainians along the Ottoman front.

The fires revealed how easily the attention of the court could be diverted from the ongoing disasters. The government had a model of how to distract and dissemble. The plague was a setback to the improvements to the health of the empire achieved by Catherine's government. Thomas Dimsdale's publications and public commemorations of his accomplishments lost value during the plague. The Academy of Sciences launched a major expedition in 1770, both designed to recapture the interest of a scientists and naturalists like the Second Kamchatka Expedition had done and to support Russia's continuing interest in exploiting its natural resources, but the restrictions on commerce imposed from plague quarantines in 1771 revealed how easily Russia's achievements could be halted. The government could still take credit for improving the health of the empire in the 1760s, but the 1770s began with a demonstration of Russia's unhygienic dangers.

The plague may have been alarming, but it did not become an obstacle for the government's intention to make progress on its health challenges. The academy's expedition gathered more evidence about the risks of, and potential solutions to, Russia's endemic diseases—scurvy, syphilis, and smallpox. Russia's ultimately successful response to controlling the plague was offered as a new guidance for other countries to adopt, and its physicians published their promising quarantine strategies. Although both were positive turns, Russia's extreme climate still offered troubling revelations. New research on the effects of cold followed, as Russia invested in solving its greatest danger. Rethinking the impact of the climate on Russian health created an opportunity to move beyond the empire's critics and even conventional knowledge about medicine: could the climate offer distinct opportunities? The immediate challenge of a pandemic could be addressed, but the long-term struggle for the health of the public continued.

The Plague

During the Russo-Turkish War (1768–1774), the bubonic plague arrived along the front between the two empires, affecting Moldova and Wallachia in 1769. Russia's physicians blamed the Ottomans for spreading the malady. In 1770, the plague arrived in Poland and Ukraine, reaching Kyiv by the summer. By November 1770, patients with plague-like symptoms were recorded in Moscow's military hospital, but it would not be until March 1771 before the Senate acknowledged that the plague had indeed arrived in Russia.[3] Charles de Mertens, a German physician working at the Moscow Foundling Hospital, recorded the arrival of the plague and its spread, symptoms, potential treatments, and preventative measures in a short tract published in Latin in 1778, in French in 1784, and in English in 1799.[4] A plague outbreak in Russia was hardly unprecedented, but one had not occurred since the 1730s. What might have been more devastating in the 1770s was that this outbreak followed Russia's significant investment in improving the empire's health. All the good work of Catherine's government was undone seemingly overnight.

Following the plague, Mertens's account was the only text written by a physician working in Russia that circulated throughout Europe. Mertens's version of events, however, was but one man's view, and this was a later version than the contemporaneous one permeating the court in St. Petersburg. The diplomats in the city closely noted the progress of the disease and kept foreign capitals abreast of the latest development. If the plague became widespread, it not only threatened Russia but also threatened all of Europe through Russia's trade connections. On April 1, 1771, news of a disease spreading in Moscow arrived in St. Petersburg. As the British ambassador extraordinary, Charles Cathcart, reported "A very ugly, malignant, if not pestilential, Fever, has broke out at Moscow; but the Court [confirms] it is not the Plague, & their Opinion seems confirm'd by the Letters the Merchants receive[d] from thence." Cathcart had learned that the fever had been transmitted in "Bales of Wool, brought from distant Parts of the Ukraine." Even if no one in St. Petersburg believed this fever was the plague, evidence indicated that this was more serious than a seasonal illness. Cathcart discovered that "there was another Alarm of this sort, some Months ago, which proceeded from the want of Care in an Hospital at Moscow, & I flatter myself, from the best Accounts I can learn, their Disorder is of the same Sort."[5] Less than a week after his initial report, Cathcart wrote with confidence, that "all apprehensions with respect to the pestilential quality of the Fever at Moscow were at an End," as he had been informed by Count Panin, and Panin's report "is since confirm[ed] from all hands."[6]

Having been assured by those at the highest level of government that the pestilential illness had ended, it is not a surprise that the fires that broke out in St. Petersburg in May were of greater concern to Cathcart than a search for other evidence about the potential plague. Moscow's continuing struggles to contain the plague, in fact, were not mentioned in court until the end of August, because the entire interest of the city was engaged first by suspected arson, and then by a more immediate illness, that of Grand Duke Paul, heir to the throne. Paul suffered from a cold that was thought to be relatively minor when it began, but, once he was not able to travel to the Peterhof Palace outside of St. Petersburg in late June, it was clear that it was more severe. On June 28, 1771, Cathcart wrote to the foreign secretary with the good news that "tho' his Imperial Highness has had a longer Continuance of this Cold than was expected when I wrote last, he has had so much better nights and symptoms so much more favourable yesterday and to day, that there is not the smallest Reason to apprehend that his Disorder will be of any Duration."[7] A distant problem in Moscow was not nearly as engrossing as the potential of Russia losing its heir.

A week after Cathcart's initial report, further details arrived from the court. Panin informed Cathcart that Paul was "as well as . . . can possibly be expected." Into the second week of a poorly-defined illness that kept the grand duke incapable of leaving his bed, interest was great for a plausible explanation. It was "thought principally to have proceeded from a Revolution in his Constitution at this time," as he had "of late grown extremely fast."[8] As Paul failed to improve throughout the summer, further explanations and optimistic predictions were offered to offset concerns. On July 5, Cathcart wrote with the expectation that "having resisted so well, so violent, and continued a Disorder, after which he will probably enjoy a firmer state of Health than before." Paul's only real challenge was that he remained confined to his bed, "and in very warm weather," which had "greatly weakened him, but he is thought to have given Proofs of an excellent Constitution."[9]

When Paul reached his third week still in bed with a fever, Cathcart began to question this optimism. Believing that "those about the Grand Duke" seem to have "a sort of Blindness" to reality, Cathcart admitted to the foreign secretary "that his situation is not without great Danger." After twenty-days days, the fever appeared to break, "which gave him Relief; but his Fever is not entirely gone; he is much troubled with a Cough, which is a late Symptom, & extremely weak & emaciated. There seems to be some hidden cause, which Nature is desirous to throw off, & if She cannot succeed, I am afraid things will end ill for him." The case was serious enough that Catherine's personal physician, Dr. John Rogerson, avoided treating the grand duke. Cathcart believed this "very lucky for that Gentlemen," as Rogerson would avoid the blame if Paul died.[10] Following this dire report, however, Paul's recovery progressed. By July 12, nearly a month after his fever began, he was "certainly better than he had been." His physicians attributed the improvement to "the late Change in the weather, which had for some time been unusually sultry."[11] On July 15, the court celebrated Paul's first day "entirely without Fever." His physicians optimistically reported his "Distemper" was "entirely over, but the Recovery from Fevers of that Duration is always extreamely slow."[12]

By the end of July, Paul had recovered sufficiently to be able to "sit up some part of the day" and was "entirely free from all his Complaints."[13] It would be months before he resumed his regular life in the court. The explanations offered at the time provide a window into medical knowledge in Russia in the 1770s. The illness was attributed to his growth spurt, which led to an imbalance of his humors. The length of his illness was affected by the climate, as proven not only by the length of the fever but also by its abatement when the weather cooled. Pharmaceutical interventions were rejected, as the "Distemper must [be] left to go off by degrees."[14] The lengthy illness in fact was a net positive for Paul, as "his Imperial Highness's Constitution will after his Recovery receive infinite advantage."[15]

The popular explanation of Paul's illness circulating in St. Petersburg would have been a greater concern for the government than the diplomatic gossip. Once news of his illness spread in the city, "the common People took the Alarm, suspected he was poisoned; and, it is said, accused very high Persons." As his illness continued for weeks, "it was given out that he was a State Prisoner, and many Officers and Under Officers of the Guards were heard to complain, that they daily expected to be called out, and if so, could not determine themselves whom they ought to obey." Catherine and Panin both rejected any suggestion of danger, but Cathcart feared that "from these Seeds someone or other much Mischief may grow."[16]

Although the court accepted the humoral explanation of the physicians, the city's populace did not. This view reflects the acceptance of humoral diagnoses that dominated literate circles, even outside the physicians in court and the naturalists at the academy. This does not mean the timing of Paul's illness was not helpful for the government in terms of distracting the court, the diplomats, and even St. Petersburg's merchants from the reality of the plague expanding in Moscow during the summer of 1771. In Mertens's later account, he confirmed the court's narrative that the plague had ended in the spring, making it unnecessary to discuss. Mertens's argument was the combination of the earlier quarantine measures in Moscow, supported by the weather remaining "very cold until the middle of April," which allowed the plague to become "fixed and inactive."[17] After all, cold temperatures had long been known to eliminate the plague.[18] Mertens, unlike Panin and the court, knew that by the end of June, an outbreak occurred at the former quarantine hospital among its staff, followed by several cases being reported in "the suburb at Preobraginsky" at the beginning of July. From then, the plague spread rapidly, overwhelming the city. By "the middle of August, the number of deaths amounted daily to four hundred; and at the end of the same month to as many as six hundred."[19]

At the same time, the government's report in late August, provided to the British foreign secretary, presented an alternate reality: "As to the Plague at Moscow, . . . it had never existed; tho' many principal Inhabitants have deserted the Town, and the Government have from complicated reasons of Policy, established a Quarantine. The miserable Poor, the only rank affected, are exposed to the precautions of the Police which would be very ludicrous were they not extreamely tragical, and fatal to great Numbers." Most important, "the Distemper, which from a similitude of some of the Symptoms has given this alarm, draws its origin not from Egypt or Turkey but from America."[20] The American argument was essential in this narrative, as the last two plagues that affected Russia earlier in the century had both emerged from the Ottoman Empire. The ambassador's report to the foreign secretary dismissed any possible connection to the plague, arguing that this outbreak was a more common North American illness that should hardly cause any fear. Had this been truthful, the similarity of the climates between Russia's Eurasian empire and its North American reaches suggested this current outbreak was an endemic issue rather than a new epidemic. The geographic origin of a disease was highly significant in terms of whom might be infected, how they might recover, and what risks foreigners could face.

Within a month, however, further news from Moscow destroyed the optimistic claim of North American origins: "that the Distemper at Moscow, tho it still has been confined to the lowest class of Inhabitants whose way of life frequently produced infections, and malignant Fevers, appears by the last accounts, even by the Letters of a private correspondent of mine who has from the beginning seen many of the sick and Dead, and never before was convinced of it, is an acknowledged and confirmed Plague."[21] For the rest of the empire, a strict quarantine had been imposed, resulting in "that unhappy City is cut off from all that Surrounds it." Even more hopeful, the country "very soon expect[s] that the front, the great Enemy to the progress of the Distemper, will set it." On the basis of these positive developments, Cathcart assured the British foreign secretary there would not be any reason to interfere with Russia's exports. The Russian government's only concern was that a "Pannick had seized the Highest as well as the lowest," leading to rioting in Moscow. Even this development was already being addressed, as Count Fedor Grigoreevich Orlov was dispatched to prosecute the rioters and restore order to the city.[22]

Catherine's government issued an *ukaz* to provide Orlov the authority to seize control over Moscow. The *ukaz* instructed the residents that Catherine acted from "maternal Condolence [for] the shocking Effects of Disease which have spread and raged in Moscow." Part of Orlov's mission was to uncover the truth of the illness, as "all Moscow will agree with me that the wide Contagion of the Distemper proceeded mostly from a false Opinion formed by a great part, nay by most, of the Inhabitants, that the Evil was not so pernicious, so infelicitous, that the Deaths ensuring from it were casual, or according to the unsearchable Will of Heaven." Once the "true cause" was known, all available resources would be provided to "stop the destructive Infection, and restore the publick Welfare." A copy of the *ukaz* was provided to Cathcart to ensure that the British government would be aware of Russia's response to eradicating the disease.[23]

From Moscow, Orlov began to update Cathcart directly. Although Cathcart's regular informant on Russian matters was Panin, Britain's trade with Russia was sufficiently important to the Russian government for immediate updates to be valuable to both parties. Orlov's first dispatch, however, was "very melancholy."[24] It was an official accounting of the recent plague riots. According to the dispatch, once the archbishop "ordered a favourite wonder-working Picture to be taken down," it inspired a quick response: "The People took the Alarm, cried out the Archbishop was robbing the Church, & guilty of Sacriledge; They rang their great Bells, assembled in great Numbers, march'd to the criminal, storm'd the Archbishop's Palace, destroyed all that was in it, except the contents of his cellars, which They drank, but did not find him, as he had sped to a Monastery at Eight Versts distance." It was only a temporary refuge, "In the Morning, They march'd to the Monastery, where They found the Archbishop celebrating Mass, They waited 'till it was over, & even 'till he had consecrated a Priest, after which, They tore him from the Sanctuary, & put him cruelly to Death by Blows given at considerable Intervals." Having killed the archbishop, the mob "destroyed all the Pest-Houses of the Police, turn'd out the Patients, swore Destruction to all Phisicians, Surgeons, &c. and buried the dead in Greek Churches. A Body of Troops was march'd against Them. They stoned the commanding Officer; They were then fired upon, & dispers'd after some Hundreds were kill'd."[25] As concerning as the deaths resulting from the riot may have been, Orlov's assessment on the current status of the plague was good news, at least for the elites and merchants: "The single symptom which is at all favorable is, that the Distemper still continues to affect only the lowest class of People, which looks as if the Air were not yet infected, & that those who live better, & keep Themselves clean are not in Danger."[26] Aside from the casual disregard for the massive loss of life resulting from the plague, Orlov suggested the lack of transmission through the air and the importance of hygiene for avoiding infection—risks elites could avoid.

Following Orlov's dispatch, Catherine led a significant effort to prevent any European response to Russia's contagion. She read Orlov's latest dispatches in court, on the principle that there was nothing to hide and to assure the public that the situation was well in hand. Immediately following Orlov's arrival in the city, he found "every thing perfectly quiet, and that the Mortality was sensibly decreased." Having observed that "many recover even in the common Hospitals, there is great reason to hope that the Distemper is past its Height and will as usual gradually diminish, especially as the weather grows colder."[27] Despite the good news from Moscow, further information arrived in St. Petersburg noting the spread of the plague to the nearby towns, which raised questions about the effectiveness of the quarantine. This news was sufficiently alarming that Cathcart suggested to the foreign minister his concern that "the Plague will not only depopulate Moscow, but several of the most fertile, & flourishing Provinces of Russia, before it can be suppress'd."[28] Catherine's strategy to allay fears may not have succeeded.

In Catherine's private correspondence with Voltaire, she did not admit that it was the plague. She acknowledged that "Disease is rife at Moscow," but "there is an epidemic of various fevers, which are causing numerous fatalities, despite all the precautions that have been taken." In her letter, she remarked that "Orlov asked as a favour to be allowed to go there [Moscow], to ascertain on the spot what measures would be the most suitable for checking the outbreak." The actual problem overtaking Moscow was not the "various fevers," but rather the residents of the city, who demonstrated the "contradictions and excesses it [the public] is capable of."[29] The violence against the archbishop, not the disease, was causing damage.

Although the Russian government remained publicly optimistic about their control over the disease, by November, both Great Britain and the Netherlands imposed quarantines on ships arriving with Russian goods. Cathcart attempted to persuade the foreign secretary these actions were unnecessary, as there had been "the least Hazard of the Plague's being brough to any of the Russian Sea Ports." Cathcart argued from what he learned from Russia's actions, no quarantine on goods was necessary. He was "assured that the Plague is not infectious unless from Contact, or from the Breadth of an Infected Person," and there had been no evidence of it spreading through "Bale goods," but he admitted it had been spread by "Cloaths which have been worn, or handled by people who are infected." Cathcart in fact seemed impressed at the methods employed by the Russian government to protect the public. If plague was discovered, the infected space was "aired, and perfumed with Vinegar, Juniper, Feathers, &c. a room set a part for any of the Family who falls ill, and who is sent to the Lazaret, if his Distemper proves to be the Plague." While the medical response impressed, the civil regulations were concerning: "The Police are generally so oppressive that poor People often chuse rather to die without assistance than to declare themselves ill, and the living are frequently so covetous that they will willfully sell or wear the Cloaths of the infected Dead and keep their apparel."[30] According to Cathcart's understanding, the high mortality in Moscow was not the result of inadequate medical care but rather oppressive policing.

By the end of the year, Cathcart responded to specific inquiries from London about the nature of the disease. The most important fact began his letter: "There is no Doubt that the Moscow Distemper is the true Levant Plague, that it has spread to so many places in the Neighborhood and to many Towns upon the Volga, and that altho' it seems to be almost every where extinguished and will so for the present be universaly and entirely so, there is great danger that by Cloaths, Furniture, and Merchandize, and by Persons, should the Distemper appear again when the Weather grows warm, the Infection may be carried, unless prevented, to the Sea Ports of Russia."[31] Cathcart had faith in the quarantine and health measures adopted by the Russian government to control the future spread of the disease, but he admitted that if "any Civil or Military Officer should suffer himself to be corrupted or surprized, Goods might pass from infected placed and might avoid the Quarantine."[32] Cathcart detailed over a series of pages the manifold steps taken to guarantee that all trade goods were properly aired and cleaned before being packed into British ships, but little of this allayed concerns about Russian officials accepting bribes to risk the public's health. Much like his earlier dispatch, the public health measures in place would be effective, if the human error of corrupt government could be avoided. When Catherine's government issued a new *ukaz* in January 1772 to protect Russia's trade goods, Cathcart dutifully sent a translation to London, but the legal protections did not alter his assessment.[33]

Despite Cathcart's fears, by the time of the January *ukaz*, the plague was under control. The Russian government was sufficiently encouraged by the effectiveness of its health measures that it prepared a guidebook for preventing the plague and even provided Cathcart a copy for the British government. The "Recipe for a fumigation powder against the plague invented for the Moscow Commission, 1771" included both the formula for the powder and an outline of nine steps for its effective use over a variety of spaces, products, and people. The powder was composed of juniper branches and berries, guaiac bark, myrrh, saltpeter, sulfur, and wheat. It was most effective when the powder was placed on burning coals in an enclosed room.[34] As evidence of its effectiveness, Cathcart relayed a report from Orlov concerning a recent experiment. Orlov "ordered, toward the End of the last year, ten malefactors who were under Sentence of Death for having been concerned in the Moscow Riot, to be confined three weeks in a Lazarette, to be laid upon the Beds, and dressed in the Cloaths, taken from men Sick, dying, and even Dead of the Plague, in the Hospital, without their having undergone any other precaution than the fumigations &c. expressed in the Paper, and none of the ten malefactors were then infected, or have since been ill."[35] Neither Cathcart nor Orlov, apparently, were concerned about the fate of ten men used in this experiment. After all, they had all been sentenced to death. We might consider death by plague to be a cruel and unusual form of punishment, but Cathcart believed it was a sensible approach to a serious issue and accepted the experiment as proof of the powder's strength.

The Russian Senate issued a new *ukaz* in March with more extensive guidelines for properly cleaning and packing trade goods to maintain exports during the quarantine.[36] With an effective prophylactic in hand, and a military presence to enforce the Senate's guidelines, the plague was under control, if not eliminated, by the spring of 1772. Concerns remained that the return of warmer weather would lead to a new outbreak, but "the going off of the Frost has produced no Symptom of Distemper any where."[37]

Cathcart's dispatches from St. Petersburg were an official account of the progress and treatment of the plague in 1771 and 1772. He reported the latest news from Catherine, Orlov, and Panin, and he had the official *ukazy* translated and dispatched. He explained in detail the current quarantine methods and included the formula for Russia's new fumigating powder. By contrast, the best-known account of the plague in Europe by the end of the century was that of Mertens. Mertens was in Moscow during the plague and had gained a reputation for his prophylactic measures, because his Foundling Hospital avoided an outbreak unlike what was experienced at the other Moscow institutions. Mertens later assessment, however, also raised some questions about what, exactly, had occurred in Moscow. He noted a broad range of symptoms, from simple headaches to visible buboes, and from mild perspiration to uncontrollable fevers. Although the buboes were the pathognomonic sign of the plague, what happened to the other patients? Indeed, Mertens recorded weeks of debate among the Russian medical establishment and government authorities, including the Senate, before a final decision was reached that this was the plague. His account plausibly suggested that the contagion may have been the plague and at least one other disease during the outbreak.

To be fair to the doubters, the plague was not a cold disease, so its presence would be seen as unlikely to many. Certainly, Russia's attempt to argue that this epidemic arrived from cold North America rather than the "hot" Ottoman Empire, relied on the physicians' nosological classification of diseases. It was beneficial to properly identify the disease as the plague, because this gave Russia's physicians the confidence that the cold climate would stop the spread of the illness. No hot disease could survive a cold climate. Russia might not be able to mitigate the effects of scurvy in its climate, but its inclement climate offered some advantages.

Mixed Peoples

Russia's suppression of the plague in 1772 was evidence of the effectiveness of the mechanisms it could implement. Conversely, the plague outbreak only a few years after its ambitious inoculation program threatened to reveal Russia's efforts as ineffective as ever. The empire was undermined by endemic diseases and the recent epidemic. Critics still argued that the population remained low and Russia's natural resources were unexploited. Apart from the catastrophe of 1771–1772, the Academy of Sciences was still dedicated to other issues. In that vein, it launched a new Siberian expedition to identify resources and address its ongoing challenges before the plague outbreak in Moscow.

The new expedition was led by Peter Simon Pallas, a German physician with specialized botany training, who became a professor at the Russian Academy of Sciences in 1768.[38] He was accompanied by Johann Gottlieb Georgi, another German physician who later joined the academy. Each man would subsequently publish his observations, contributing toward another official record of the empire's resources; within a decade of the texts' first publications, they would appear in German, French, and English editions.[39] The expedition left St. Petersburg before the plague arrived in Moscow, but its publications followed the plague. Considering the timing of the expedition, as well as the general tasks confronting the academicians, it is no surprise that the health of the empire featured as prominently in their texts as it had in reports from the Second Kamchatka Expedition. Both Pallas and Georgi relied on earlier German naturalists' commentaries on Russia, particularly Johann Georg Gmelin's and Georg Wilhem Steller's accounts. Pallas's and Georgi's narratives, therefore, had numerous similarities, built on common precedents, and shared a purpose of providing a complete description of the people and resources of the Russian Empire. Their reliance on Gmelin and Steller resulted in significant similarities in their observations.

Georgi's volumes are the more thorough of the two, in terms of descriptions of imperial subjects. He presented each group within a continuum: a physical description of the typical man and woman as well as an examination of their lifestyles and occupations; clothing and customs (with a particular focus on marriage and childbirth); health and illness; and food, climate, and temperament. In other words, he included all of the nonnaturals. The English edition of his text, *Russia: Or A Compleat Historical Account of All of the Nations which Compose that Empire* (1780–1783), was translated by William Tooke, who was then the chaplain of the Russia Company in St. Petersburgh but would become a future member of the academy. Tooke eventually produced another comprehensive assessment of the all of the peoples of the empire, but that text would not be published until the turn of the century.[40] Georgi's

Russia envisioned the Russian Empire as a series of ethnolinguistically defined bands across the empire. It began with "Laplanders" stretching from Scandinavia across northern Russian until reaching the Ural Mountains; continued with "Tatars" as a broad Turkic group from Kazan' in the south and east until meeting the Iakuts on the border of China; and then arrived at the "Samoyeds" from the Urals in the east to Kamchatka. None of these labels works by modern conceptions of ethnolinguistic identity, including the numerous Finno-Ugric people who across the region who did not neatly fit into the Laplander and Samoyed groups.

These divisions reflect those defined by Carl Linnaeus. Skin color and geography influenced his four types of man, two of whom were readily identified in the Russian Empire. In Linnaeus's classification, the Laplanders were the white Europeans and the Tatars were "dark" Asians.[41] The challenge of Russia, and its primary contribution toward this taxonomic system, were the groups that fell between European and Asian. Tooke translated the last section of *Russia* as "Various Nations whose Origin is Mixed and Uncertain"; it was primarily the Samoyed group, composed of various Siberian populations, including some of the Ostiaks, the Tungus, and Itelemen from Kamchatka.[42] But this liminal category, spanning thousands of miles across Eurasia, highlighted some of the shortcomings of Linnaeus's system. Whatever division could be drawn between Europeans and Asians collapsed in the expanse of the Russian Empire.

This does not imply that Georgi's study did not see broad similarities across the empire. Indeed, he accepted that similar environments produced similar bodies. Most of the people of the empire were described as either phlegmatic or melancholic (i.e., the cold constitutions). The Laplanders, those Finnic peoples on the northwestern edge of the empire, for example, were "of a middling stature. They have generally a flattish face, fallen cheeks, dark grey eyes, thin beard, brown hair, are well-built, straight, and of a yellowish complexion, occasioned by the weather." Laplander women were "short, complaisant, chaste, often well-made, and extremely nervous." Both sexes in Georgi's description were portraits of phlegmatic complexion, including chasteness, as disinterest in sexual activity was another phlegmatic sign. It follows a humoral logic, therefore, that "venereal disease is unknown in Lapland." In spite of this disinterest, perhaps, Laplanders did procreate. "Sterility is a sort of reproach among the Lapland women, . . . They are generally delivered without difficulty. The husband assists at the labour, and affords his wife the necessary help. Without this practice they would often be distressed, as the habitations are frequently at such a distance one from another to preclude the aid of any other women." Childbirth was not their only challenge, as "their common diseases are the itch, phthisis, and putrid fevers. They are subject to inflammations in the eyes, the effects of the snow and the continual smoke they are exposed to in their huts."[43]

The Laplanders compared poorly to their neighbors, the Finns. They were a "fertile stock," and more important, Finns were "the parent of almost all the northern nations of Europe," although they were "of Asiatic origin." The Finns "lived to a very advanced age; although the dropsy, the scurvy, the epilepsy, . . . are disease very common among the country people." The Estonians were "very like the Finns. Great numbers of them are of a phlegmatic and melancholic disposition. Except life itself, and the pleasures of love, every thing in the world is indifferent to them." Primarily, he concluded, the phlegmatic nature made them "idle, filthy, and addicted to drunkenness." Many of the broad "Laplander" group faced similar criticism. Mari "men have neither the vivacity nor the determined character of the Russians; and their women are much inferior to those of Russia, as well in regard to comeliness, as in gaiety of temper, and vanity of dress." The Chuvashes "have indeed a paler complexion, are more lazy, and are not so sharp-witted" as the Maris. Georgi and Tooke frequently described the humoral bodies of the imperial subjects in these types of stereotypical strokes. The "Barabintzes," a Turkic group living on the Baraba steppe south of Ufa, were "almost all of them of a phlegmatic habit, with a pale complexion, to which natural dullness may be added to their poverty and want of instruction." This was the result of "the air of Baraba during the summer [which] is continually charged with vapour." The poor climate of Baraba was such that they were "cold even in their amours, and rarely drink to intoxication."[44]

Considerable effort was given to documenting marriage rituals and birth practices across the empire. This reflected the ongoing concern with raising the empire's birth rates, an effort that had begun more than a decade earlier. The Mordvins of the Middle Volga Region, for example, "when the time of delivery approaches, the women retire to the bathing room. Here she receives the accustomed visits, and those of her friends, who name the new-born child." Among the Nogai Tatars on the southern steppe, "their manner of facilitating, as they call it, the delivery of their women, is exactly contrary to common sense; when the women is near her time they tie a belt under her arms, by which they

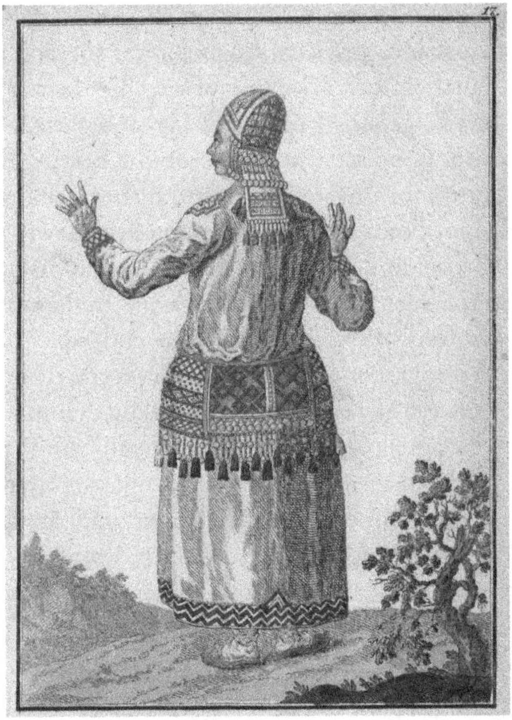

Figure 5.1. Georgi's illustration of a Mordvin woman. "Finskie narody: Mordovka so spinoiu," Rare Book Division, The New York Public Library, New York Public Library Digital Collections, accessed June 9, 2024, https://digitalcollections.nypl.org/items/19ef0b30-c6d2-012f-72ae-58d385a7bc34.

hoist her up and let her fall successively" (figure 5.1). Among the Samoyeds of Siberia, "women are delivered with surprising facility, almost without pain or any accident; the least pain in child-birth causes an immediate suspicion that she has had some illicit conversation with other men, and therefore is let to suffer, for the sake of extorting a confession of her fault, with the name of her gallants, who, in such a case, may save themselves trouble of any justification, as, whether innocent or guilty, they must make satisfaction to the injured husband; but these reparations consist almost always in some trifle."[45]

The Samoyeds were hardly alone in their concern over potential infidelities; Georgi documented a range of reactions across the empire. For the Tatars of Kazan', Georgi argued that the Quran inspired their social mores, as it "allows polygamy, so that the faithful take no more than four wives; who all enjoy the same rights, having each a claim to the caresses of the husband in turn." If "one of these wives follows amorous intrigues," her husband "gives her up to the gallant, and takes to himself another." Furthermore, "the loss of virginity before these proper preliminaries [marriage] being reckoned a great reproach, a young husband who does not mind secrecy on this, on not finding the testimonials thereof the next morning, or by pretending not to have found them, may by this means obtain an augmentation of the dower from the parents." Finally, Georgi noted that "sterility is a great disgrace to a wife, especially when the husband has more than one; in that case, the barren woman is always despised by those who have children."[46]

This is not to imply that Georgi ignored venereal disease, but it was only a minor concern if mentioned at all. For example, the Ostiaks "have a flattish face of a pale yellow colour, harsh hair of a deep colour, a thin beard, a dull understanding, and a phlegmatic temperament; consequently, they are timorous, superstitious, and lazy, dirty and disgusting; but tractable, mild and a good-hearted people." Despite their phlegmatic temperament in a cold environment, the Ostiaks did "enjoy a good state of health, but as soon as old age obliges them to stay within doors, they are much afflicted with the scurvy, the itch, and inflammations of the eyes. . . . The venereal disease is very common with them. In every kind of disorder, as soon as they fell themselves affected they burn their skin till it cracks; to produce this effect they use a fungus found on the birch-trees, which they call *yagbani*" (figure 5.2). Applying a local cure to treat venereal diseases was a humoral solution to the problem. Similarly, the Kirghiz enjoyed a "manner of life, simple, natural, and except from care, joined to the pure air of their vast and open deserts, preserves them from divers diseases, and numbers of them arrive at an extreme old age, hearty and full of vivacity. The indispositions to which they are most subject are the itch, coughs, and agues. Some are attacked by venereal disease." In Georgi's description, both the Ostiaks and Kirghiz reached an advanced age despite these common diseases, which indicated that the earlier anxiety about procreation and venereal disease was unnecessary. The only disease that Georgi suggested endangered the empire was smallpox, which "made great havoc amongst" the Ostiaks and committed "great ravages" to the Kirghiz.[47] Because Georgi wrote his narrative after Catherine's inoculation program began, his text arguably highlighted progress against syphilis, which did not cause serious issues in his narrative, and smallpox, which did but was being addressed.

In southern Russia, a temperate climate appropriately produced more active men and women, with some becoming sanguine or choleric.

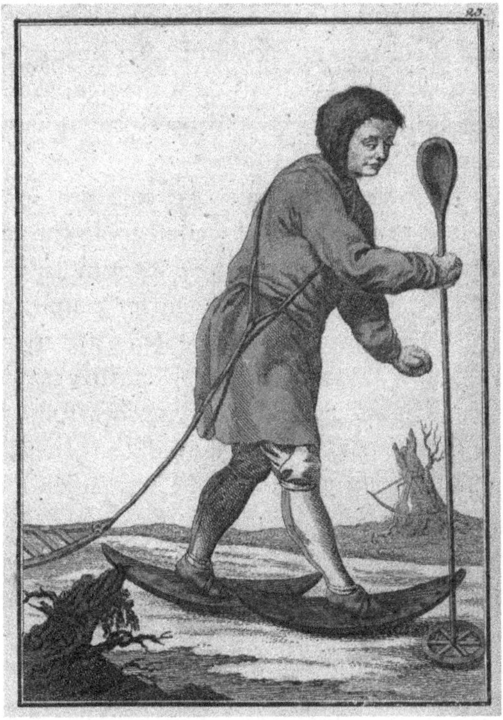

FIGURE 5.2. Georgi's illustration of an Ostiak man hunting an ermine. "Finskie narody: Ostiak na lovle gornostaev," Rare Book Division, The New York Public Library. New York Public Library Digital Collections, accessed June 9, 2024, https://digitalcollections.nypl.org/items/510d47df-c182-a3d9-e040-e00a18064a99.

The "warm climate" of the Caucasus featured people who engaged in commerce, and those in agriculture produced crops for the market. The Kalmyks were "a mixture of sanguine and phlegmatic, the melancholy is seldom uppermost. They have a good understanding, and a quick comprehension, . . . [are] sprightly, hospitable, ready to do kind offices, active and voluptuous." As a result of their healthy temperament, they knew "but little of sickness." A group like the Baraba Tatars reflected the challenge of the cold, whereas other groups from the southern climes avoided their implicit weakness. The Bukharans, for example, enjoyed a "fine climate no less favourable to Venus than to Bacchus. A man tolerably at his ease takes two wives, and several have three or four. It is not, therefore, without reason, that both sexes use an infusion of *salab* [orchid root] as frequently as other nations take coffee. The invigorating and stimulating properties of that root are less equivocal in Bougharia than they are in colder regions. They roast them at the fire, then reduce them to a powder, and, after having poured boiling water on them, they drink the infusion with sugar exactly as we take coffee."[48] For Georgi, the connection between environment and sexual activity was clear.

Any analysis of lifestyle applied to the cold peoples of Russia, or the few hot peoples in the far south, fell apart in the eastern regions of the empire. The division between the European Laplanders and the Asian Tatars failed to accommodate the mixed peoples of Siberia and Kamchatka. The Tungus, for example, were of a "very sanguine constitution, frank, and always appear to be what they really are. . . . They feel no disquietude about the morrow, but chearfully divide the last morsel with the first comer, and the gaiety of the conversation is never diminished by the indigence of the host." Their sanguine temperament was not without its flaws, of course, as they could fly into a "rage" over "the merest trifles." According to Georgi, "These nomads, hardy, sober, active, free from care, are acquainted with few diseases, and have none peculiar to themselves, yet they never live to a very advanced age." He argued that the cause of death was most often "the scurvy, from want of that exercise which they have continually been used from their infancy. A several small-pox has now and then appeared among them."[49] Russian authorities would have likely preferred to avoid further mentions of the endemic nature of scurvy and smallpox, the two diseases most often mentioned in the empire, but this also reflected the mixed bodies of the Tungus (figure 5.3). Their complexion was sanguine, but they still suffered from the most famous cold disease of all, scurvy. The disease was predictable based on their environment and diet, but it was also proof of the difficulty of fitting these specific people into a restrictive system—either Linnaeus's taxonomy or traditional humoral assessments.

Georgi's "Kamchadals" also offered contradictions. Explicitly relying on Steller's history of Kamchatka, Georgi noted "their immoderate lust proceeds even to bestiality; and the men, contrary to the custom of other eastern nations, make themselves the voluntary slaves of the women to gratify their lascivious desires. Pederasty is practiced almost publicly." The cause of this wantonness was "their daily use of half-rotten fish, fish-roe, rancid fat, and onions; but especially to their excessive indolence." The Kamchadals were an "eastern" people who were "strong and healthy," which were hot qualities. Like the Tungus, however, it was scurvy that plagued them. Unlike the Tungus, they also suffered from endemic venereal disease, which Georgi assured his readers

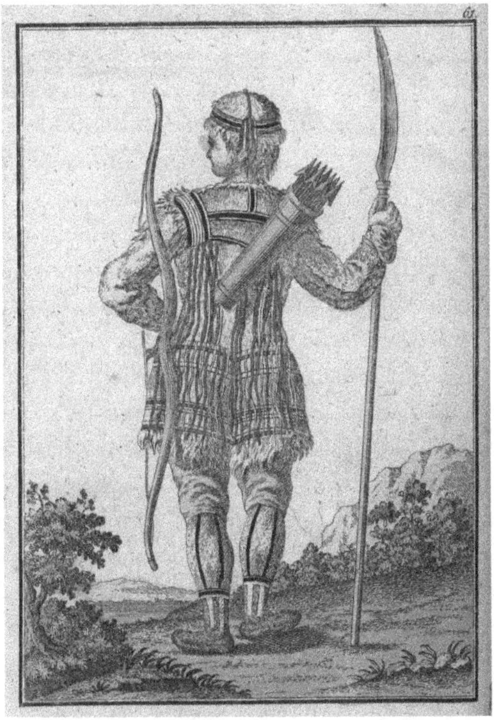

FIGURE 5.3. Georgi's illustration of a Tungus man. "Mandzhurskie narody: Tunguz v okhotnichem plat'e s tyla," Rare Book Division, The New York Public Library. New York Public Library Digital Collections, accessed June 9, 2024, https://digitalcollections.nypl.org/items/510d47df-c1a8-a3d9-e040-e00a18064a99.

"was known to them before the Russians arrived." But, more troubling, "they formerly inoculated their children for the small-pox, by scratching the face with a fish-bone dipt in variolous matter. As this distemper made no appearance for a number of years, they neglected this salutary practice, when in 1758 it was unluckily brought there by a soldier, who had been a long time cured of it. This scourge of the human race then raged in so dreadful and fatal a manner, that it swept away two thirds of the nation."[50] His assessment on the diseases served as a response to Jean-Baptiste Chappe d'Auteroche, as the Russians may have introduced smallpox, but were not responsible for its consequences as the Kamchadals had already abandoned inoculation. Nor had the Russians introduced venereal disease. Although this depiction might have served the government's interests, it did not alter the confusing bodies and climate of Kamchatka. Were these people European or Asian, hot or cold? What did it mean to be mixed?

The confusion over the possibility of mixed peoples reflected Georgi's description of the Buriats, who like the Kalmyks, were both "the sanguine and the phlegmatic." Georgi's view is appropriately full of contradictory qualities. The Buriats were "much indolent, and at the same time too great lovers of a wandering life. . . . They experience but little sickness or diseases, yet, for all that, they but seldom attain to the age of threescore years." The main challenges were smallpox, from which "great numbers die," but the Russian government recently established a new smallpox clinic in Irkutsk to inoculate them. They also were "acquainted with the venereal disease" and were frequent sufferers of "the itch," but this resulted from "their lazy and dirty way of life, and their hot fur-clothing."[51] The positive and negative qualities were presented in quick juxtaposition. This may have reflected their position between the Russian Empire and China, producing a mixed quality not seen in the empire at large. Another possibility is that because Georgi did not travel to the far eastern regions of the empire before writing his text, his reliance on earlier texts to classify this group could have created a dissonance from his otherwise distinct separation of humors and climates within the empire. For the Kamchadals, Georgi willingly relied on Steller, but for the Buriats, he never identified his informant.

Georgi's exhaustive description aspired to be a complete view of all imperial subjects, but he was not the only naturalist on the expedition. Pallas's description of imperial subjects was not as lengthy, but it drew on similar notions of cold peoples in the north, hot in the south, and it accepted some division between European and Asian bodies. At the southern edge of the empire, for example, Pallas was a great admirer of the Kalmyks, whom he described "as affable, hospitable and honest; they like to render service; they are always cheerful and gay, which distinguishes them from the Kirghiz [of Siberia], who are phlegmatic." As nomads, however, the Kalmyks did have some weaknesses, particularly "uncleanliness, which arose from their lack of education." Pallas later provided ample evidence of the Kirghizes' phlegmatic nature, as he observed that they commonly suffered from colds, asthma, heart palpitations, and venereal disease, all linked to coldness (figure 5.4). He also noted a lack of evidence that the Kirghiz suffered from fevers, although this was a common problem among the "warmer" Kalmyks.[52]

Pallas's expedition was both a summative process, compiling all the views of the German naturalists from the previous decades, and a formative one, highlighting Russia's imperial achievements and outlining

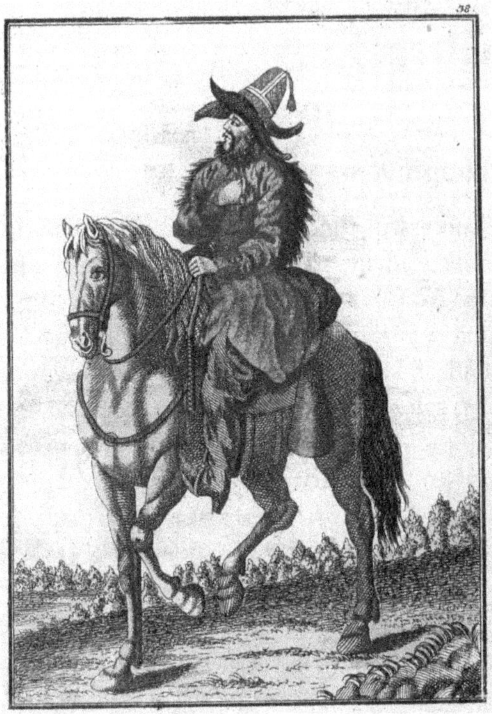

FIGURE 5.4. Georgi's illustration of a Kirghiz man on horseback. "Tatarskie narody: Kirgizets na kone," Rare Book Division, The New York Public Library, New York Public Library Digital Collections, accessed June 9, 2024, https://digitalcollections.nypl.org/items/510d47df-c190-a3d9-e040-e00a18064a99.

necessary interventions for further improvements. Georgi had a deep interest in increasing the size of the population; investigating marriage and birth rituals, sexual activities, and the pervasiveness of venereal diseases; and identifying the leading causes of mortality for every group in the empire. This process underscored the persistent challenge of scurvy, smallpox, and syphilis across the empire. Georgi not only noted those places where the state made inroads to controlling smallpox but also revealed how limited those efforts were across the empire. As the Second Kamchatka Expedition's records did, this information provided ammunition both for Russia's advocates and its critics. The extensive details about mixed peoples, who were neither European nor Asian, however, challenged Linnaeus's classification schema. Russia's contribution to human taxonomy was to complicate its categories, at a moment when European ideas of race as a fixed category were influencing colonial decisions in the Atlantic world.[53] Highlighting the ways in which Russia's imperial subjects were exceptional served as a critique of the taxonomic system that had become increasingly dominant.

Institutional Improvements

Following the successful conclusion of Pallas's expedition, it was once again time for the academy to celebrate its achievements. Pallas's third and final volume from his expedition was published in 1776, and later that same year it was the fiftieth anniversary of the Academy of Sciences. At the end of 1776, the academy held a congratulatory jubilee with all the court's dignitaries. Grand Duke Paul and his new wife were in attendance, and a series of speeches were offered in their honor from both the director and secretary of the academy. In addition, "His Imperial Highness & the King of Prussia were inscribed Members of the Academy and several Natives and Foreigners of great Eminence in different Branches of Knowledge were likewise received into that learned Body. Medals struck upon this Occasion, and a new Map of the Russian Empire, were presented to their Imperial Highnesses." Three days later, on January 1, 1777, "there was a brilliant and numerous Court in the morning when the foreign Ministers had the Honour of paying their Compliments to the Empress, and the Members of the Academy of Sciences were presented to Her Imperial Majesty."[54]

Arguably, the academy and its members had notable successes in the fifty years of its existence. The plague arriving hard upon the heels of the smallpox inoculation campaign beginning did not undo Russia's progress in terms of improving the empire's health, but Russia's critics were not silent. There is no doubt that Britain and its diplomats continued to protest, but, as always, they kept their complaints among the diplomatic corps rather than as public knowledge. French *philosophes*, however, continued to depict Russia as a demonstration of failure. The economist Marbault, for example, argued that the Russians were continually endangered by the "poor food and excessive cold," which added to the "physical deprivations of poverty, servitude, and the violence employed to force them work" produced rampant scurvy, which the use of the bania failed to cure. Russia's only chance for success was that Russian women were "the most fertile" in Europe, regularly having "ten children."[55] When Georgi published his multivolume *Russia* in 1779, the extensive details on birth rates among all groups in the empire responded to Marbault's claim, but there was no question Russia's critics still pointed to reproductive shortcomings and endemic diseases as evidence of Russia's inability to manage its subjects and climate.

Russia's Academy of Sciences and its College of Medicine continued to strive to improve health outcomes for the population. It is true that both the Second Kamchatka Expedition and Pallas's expedition highlighted the endemic nature of scurvy, syphilis, and smallpox in Siberia. With Dimsdale's inoculation campaign begun in 1768, the state would make inroads against one of these diseases, but the others remained uncontrolled. The academy was continuously gathering information for the treatment of scurvy, but there was yet no single fix to this classic cold illness. The state's agents, however, had barely addressed venereal disease. As a result, developing a therapy for treatment of this ongoing threat allowed Catherine's government to formulate at least one response to the negative publicity that followed their pandemic eruptions.

In 1776, the academy published its first text on the treatment of the "French Pox" (*frantsuzskaia bolezniia*) by S. A. Venechanskii.[56] Venechanskii explicitly linked the importance of this text to the state's demographic concerns, as noted at the beginning that "the first to be infected by this disease are childbearing women." At the same time, from a modern perspective, it is not always clear which disease Venechanskii believed the French disease to be, as he observed that it had "varied symptoms, affects different parts of the body, and is known by many names."[57] This is not to be critical of his knowledge, debates were ongoing across Europe about syphilis and the other venereal diseases. On the positive side, he took a broad view of the possible origins for the disease, its transmission, and its symptoms, providing information for potentially diagnosing a wider array of ailments than might be expected. Approximately one-third of the text focused on the various remedies that could be prepared for the disease (or diseases), with more than twenty options, although most involved some amount of mercury, including in two "Neopolitan" salves and one attributed to physicians in Venice.

Venechanskii's text was not the only information available to Russia's physicians. Two years later, A. G. Bakherakht published *On Immoderation of the Passions of Both Sexes* (1778). His central argument was that successful childrearing should instill moral fiber to prevent venereal disease.[58] The majority of Bakherakht's work was on the health of Russia's navy. Venereal disease was primarily a military issue rather than a demographic one as in Venechanskii's work, so the different solution to the issue was not simply a moral versus medical one. These two texts, however, are the only Russian-language ones that addressed venereal disease in the eighteenth century, and thus Russia lacked the array of medical opinions on the subject common across Europe. For comparison, more than three hundred pamphlets and books on venereal disease were published in Britain in the seventeenth and eighteenth centuries.[59] This fact, however, fails to account for the reality that the overwhelming majority of physicians in Russia were either German, British, or Russian Empire-born and German educated. Therefore, these physicians had access to both German and English-language texts on the subject. Venechanskii and Bakherakht's texts in Russian were part of the turn toward making more information available to surgeons and apothecaries, moving potential treatment for venereal disease to a broader group than just the specialist, foreign-trained physicians.

The College of Medicine was no less invested in improving the health of the empire than the academy's specialists were. In particular, the college made an investment in increasing the number of hospitals providing care in the major cities. When the English minister and traveler William Coxe visited the empire in 1778, he was impressed with these institutions. The one receiving his greatest appreciation was the Foundling Hospital in Moscow. Its fame had been established by its escape from infection during the plague earlier in the decade. When he visited, it held three hundred orphans, although it planned to hold eight hundred. Coxe was impressed by its overall efficiency. All children were welcomed, and immediately registered and baptized. Then "the child is first visited by a surgeon before it is carried into the house: it is new-clothed, and given to a wet nurse, there being always a certain number attending for that purpose. A wet nurse never suckles more than one child." The children were managed by age and ability throughout their years in the hospital. Before the age of seven, all of the children were kept together to "learn to read, write, and cast accounts." After that, they were kept in separate wards, where the "boys are taught knitting; they occasional card hemp, flax, and wool, and are sooner or later employed in the different manufacturers." Separately, "the girls learn to knit, net, and all kinds of needle-work. They spin and weave lace; they are taught cookery, baking; and are employed in house-work of all sorts." After fourteen, both boys and girls worked different rooms to learn particularly trade skills, including embroidery or furniture construction, and then they were finally released at twenty in expectation they would be able to support themselves.[60] It was providing twenty years of "support" that most impressed Coxe, but for thirteen of those years, the orphans were actually supporting themselves in this workhouse.

Coxe also admired Moscow's Imperial Hospital; it had been established by Peter the Great as Russia's primary medical facility for injured soldiers. It was a brick building "in a very airy situation," with two main wards for 120 patients each, which were long and broad and had high spaces. One was designated for patients with fevers, and the other for "chiefly scorbutic and wounded." It also held special rooms designated for venereal patients. "The chambers for venereal disease were in outhouses; one room with seventy-five beds contained seventy-three patients."[61] It was clear that the venereal patients, kept in small rooms outside the main facility ("outhouses"), were not considered to be a part of the wounded and ill in the public spaces of the hospital. Although Coxe mentioned several other hospitals in Moscow, none of the others contained a separate space for venereal patients, suggesting venereal disease was a problem for its soldiers, at least in terms of hospital care. It should not have been a surprise that of the three primary spaces for patients at the hospital, two were focused on treatments for scurvy and syphilis, the primary health challenges still confronting Russia.

Coxe believed that Russia's hospitals were first-rate institutions, but he was equally impressed by the care provided in Russia's prisons. His descriptions demonstrated the influence of the general health improvements achieved during Catherine's reign. Coxe expected evidence of "epidemical distempers" among Russia's prisoners, "but could not hear of the least tendency to such disorders." The absence of disease was a result of an effective regime imposed on the prison system. Coxe noted that "care that is taken not to over-crowd the jails; the custom which prevails of suffering the prisoners to go occasionally to the baths; the first of the prisons, which in general are built in airy situations, and almost always provided with court yards, where the prisoners are allowed to walk in the day-time." In winter, preparations were taken to mitigate "the intense cold which continues for several months together; the quass, a fermented liquor, which is reckoned a fine antiscorbutic; it is the general drink, in Russia; an rye-bread, which is also deemed a great sweetner of the blood, is their principal food. Add to this the custom of smoking the wards by burning juniper branches and berries."[62] This health regimen was a combination of lessons learned on the treatment of scurvy (particularly kvass) with the fumigation methods developed during the plague. Coxe's comments about the prisons demonstrated that the Russian government was capable of successfully implementing its solutions to its recent health struggles.

Although visitors such as Coxe praised Russia's accomplishments, the men working for Russia were no less active in documenting Russia's health interventions. One of the most prolific men writing on the topic was a Scottish physician, Matthew Guthrie, who had a long career in Russia. Guthrie was born in Edinburgh in 1743 and studied medicine at the University of Edinburgh in 1762 and 1763. Guthrie was appointed as a surgeon for the Admiralty during the Russo-Turkish War (1769–1774). By 1778, he became the chief medical officer to the Land Corps of Noble Cadets, which was a position he would hold until his death in 1807. He also became a member of Russia's Free Economic Society in 1778 and a member of the Royal Society of London in 1782. though he was not a member of the Russian Academy of Sciences, his scientific work involved experiments conducted alongside Pallas and Samuel Gottlieb Gmelin.[63]

As was the case for many of his contemporaries in Russia, Guthrie maintained an active correspondence with his colleagues in Europe, and his preferred topic was the cold climate and the endemic diseases resulting from exposure to that climate. In a letter published in *Medical and Philosophical Commentaries* in 1777, the University of Edinburgh's medical journal, he discussed local remedies for "arthritical disorders" and rheumatism, both of which he revealed as being widespread throughout Siberia. The residents of Siberia relied on a tea brewed from *Rhododendron chrysanthemum*, as "discovered by my learned friend Professor Pallas" (figure 5.5). The treatment was simple, as Siberians "take about two drams of the dried shrub, stalk and leaves, with nine or ten ounces of boiling water, and putting them into an earthen pot, they lute on the head, and place them in an oven during the nights. This infusion, for it is not allowed to boil, the sick man drinks next morning for a dose." Its effects were immediate: "It occasions heat, together with a degree of intoxication, resembling the effects of spirituous liquors, and a singular kind of uneasy sensation in the parts affected, accompanied with a sort of vermiculation, which is likewise confined to the diseased parts. The patient is not permitted to quench the thirst which this medicine occasions, as fluids, particularly cold water, produce vomiting, which lessens the power of the specific." Guthrie was optimistic about the benefits. Although he warned "that the dose which these hardy Siberians take, who are also in the habit of drinking it as tea, would, in all probability, be too strong for our

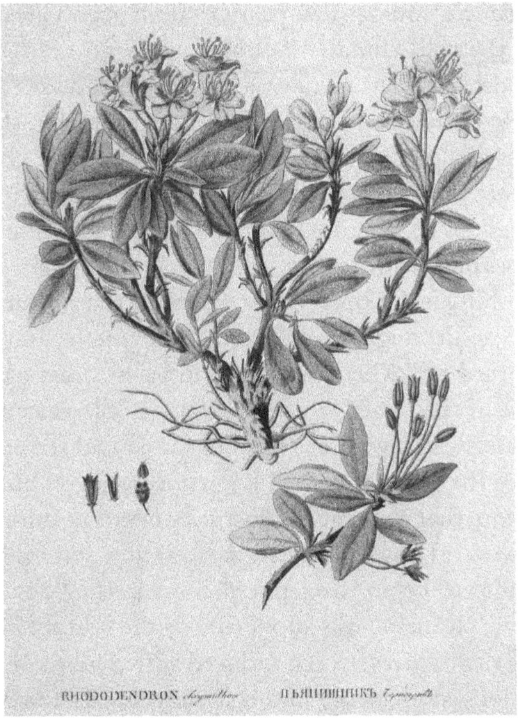

FIGURE 5.5. Pallas's illustration of *Rhododendron chrysanthemum*, from his *Flora Rossica* (1784–1788). "Rhododendron chrysanthum; P'ianishnik chernogriv," Rare Book Division, The New York Public Library, New York Public Library Digital Collections, accessed October 11, 2024, https://digitalcollections.nypl.org/items/510d47df-e84e-a3d9-e040-e00a18064a99.

countrymen; however, it is a medicine which we may certainly give with safety, beginning with small doses."[64]

The following year, in 1778, Guthrie published his first letter in *Philosophical Transactions of the Royal Society of London*, once again promoting Russian therapies for a cold disease, but this time highlighting scurvy. Guthrie's interest was in understanding how Russians avoided illness, particularly that "they must undoubtedly have sunk under the scurvy, as they are, for the greatest part of the year, exposed to the influence of those pre-disposing causes to putrid complaints that make the body of the Greenland seamen livid." As Guthrie noted, physicians still accepted that "bad air within, excessive cold without, joined to a want of fresh vegetables for a length of time" that caused putrefaction within a body, producing scurvy as its inevitable outcome.[65] Despite the conditions for illness, scurvy was largely unknown among the Russian peasantry.

Guthrie's conclusion was that peasants developed a lifestyle designed to overcome the cold climate. It first began with a diet rich in anti-scorbutic foods: sour cabbage, kvass, rye bread, and salted cucumbers. These "acidulous" foods prevented putrefaction within the body. Furthermore, Russian peasants developed "some customs" that "probably have their share in effecting" putrefaction; "these are their cloathing, baths, and manner of sleeping." Guthrie felt the clothing was perhaps the most important, with "many plies of coarse flannel, . . . sheep skin coats, and nothing is left open to the action of the air but the face and neck, which last although never covered, yet coughs and sore throats are seldom heard of." Their healthy manner of dress was supported by regular use of the bania, where Russians "wash away with aqueous vapour, and afterwards with water in its condensed state, the dirt that by obstructing the pores is so well known to promote putrid diseases, at the same time that they most effectually open the cuticular emunctories, and throw off any obstructed perspiration that might otherwise acted as a fomes to begin the septic process in the body." Ultimately, the bania's pore cleansing was supported by the peasant habit of sleeping on top of their stoves, which induced sufficient daily perspiration to undue the effects of being in a cold climate. If, however, peasants were kept "from the nocturnal luxury of their oven, and you [would] kill them in a week." Guthrie concluded his letter with a warning for his fellow foreigners living in Russia: They must abandon their "European" habits for "the experience that a succession of ages has taught the natives" about the proper way to mitigate the consequences of the climate.[66]

Guthrie's letter was followed in that volume of *Philosophical Transactions* by another physician with a career in Russia, Charles de Mertens. By 1778, however, Mertens had left Moscow's Foundling Hospital and was a professor of medicine at the University of Vienna. The same year he published his plague tract, he analyzed the treatment for scurvy, once again drawn from his career in Moscow. Mertens agreed with the conventional wisdom that scurvy was a continuing challenge for ocean voyages because of sailors' reliance on salted foods, but he commended recent experiments with mitigating the dangers with a diet that included sauerkraut. Although he did not question its effectiveness, he argued that "at Moscow, many gentlemen merchants and strangers were attacked by a slow scurvy, having their gums soft, swollen, and blueish, the breath strong, and many scorbutic spots at the legs, whilst it was rare to find among the lower people, either of town or country" despite the foreigners regularly eating "a soup made of sour cabbage, exactly resembling the German sour-krout in every thing." After years of observing this mystery, Mertens concluded that the Russians "were indebted for their safety to the great quantity of raw greens, such as onions, leeks, raddishes, turnips, peas in the pod, and others, which they eat. The berries of Vaccinum, which others much resembling them, called *kloukua*, which are of the size of a small cherry and very acid, are together with applies, strawberries, and raspberries, almost the only fruits of these countries." During a large scurvy outbreak in the Foundling Hospital during the winter of 1771, Mertens implemented this fruit and green vegetable diet, and the children rapidly recovered. In this therapeutic choice, Mertens more closely followed Steller's advice from the Second Kamchatka Expedition than Guthrie's recommendation. Mertens was explicit that the bania made little difference, because the Russians' lifestyle was "extremely nasty" compared with the "people of fashion."[67] Although Mertens wrote far less admiringly of Russians' health, he was no less impressed with the Russians' success in adapting to their environment.

Before the end of 1778, a former British resident of St. Petersburg published a pamphlet on the climate that supported Guthrie. It was written by John Glen King, who was a fellow of the Royal Society of London and had been the chaplain of the Russia Company for a decade. King's observations on the best methods to moderate the influence of the cold climate resembled Guthrie's view. King argued that while Russia's coldness was "severe, . . . it is seldom that any body suffers from it, so easy are the means and so plentiful are the provisions to guard against it." According to King, the solution was "the method of warming the houses by an oven constructed with several flues, and that the country abounds with wood, which is the common fuel."[68] King also mentioned that Russians were "cloathed so warmly they bid defiance to frost and snow," again agreeing with Guthrie's conclusions.

King added a new element to the discussion. He observed that while Russia may have been extremely cold, "the wind is never violent in winter, and in general there is very little wind," saving Russians from exposure to "cold that is exceedingly piercing." Therefore, even if "the winters seem long and tedious in these northern climates," Russians' enjoyment of snow "makes even this much more tolerable to the natives, as well as their happy ignorance of better climes." King was far kinder about summer weather, noting that then conditions "differ much less from southern climates." Even "some persons [who] reckon the light nights in summer an agreeable circumstance," benefiting from "so great a brightness one may see to read and write at midnight, unless it be cloudy, for full two months."[69]

The following year, Guthrie published another letter in *Philosophical Transactions*, perhaps responding to Mertens's implication that the Russians' lifestyle was unhealthy, not only from the climate but also from their small houses, which were dominated by a large stove. Guthrie's letter discussed how Russians recovered from inhaling "the Fumes of burning Charcoal" throughout the long winter. "Russian houses are heated by the means of ovens; . . . a number of billets of woods are placed in the peech or stove, and allowed to burn till they fall in a mass of bright red cinders; then the vent above is shut up, and likewise the door of the peech which opens into the room, in order to concentrate the heat; this makes the tiles of which the peech is composed as hot as you desire, and sufficiently warms the apartment." The stove, in turn, releases a vapor that places a person "into so sound a sleep that it is difficult to awake him, but he feels (or is sensible of) nothing." If this person has been "suffocated" by the vapor, which "seldom affects a Russian," a "recovery is always attempted." The patient is carried outdoors, and laid in the snow, "with nothing on but a shirt and linen drawers. His stomach and temples are then well rubbed with snow, and cold water, or milk is poured down his throat. This friction is continued with fresh snow until the livid hue, which the body had when brought out, is changed to its natural colour, and life renewed; then they cure the violent head-ach which remains by binding on the forehead a cataplasm of black rye bread, and vinegar." Guthrie did not offer any conclusion about whether or not the vapor was dangerous to the lungs or the circulatory system, as "I shall leave that to your investigation." He only commented that "it is so common a case here that it is perfectly familiar to them [the Russians], and they never call in medical assistance."[70] Whereas Mertens suggested Russians remained healthy despite their lifestyle, Guthrie remained far more optimistic that the Russians had successfully answered the challenges of their lives in this cold climate.

Guthrie would remain more important to the Russian medical and scientific establishment than Mertens. After all, his career lasted decades in St. Petersburg, whereas Mertens left for Vienna. Visiting Guthrie became a necessary stop for newly arrived British men in Russia's capital. Samuel Bentham, for example, arrived in Russia in the spring of 1780, carrying a variety of letters of introduction. One of those was for the British consul to Russia, Walter Shairp, who immediately introduced Bentham to Guthrie "not as a Physitian, . . . but as a friend. In a day or two Dr. Guthrie came, I found him a Man of very clear Ideas perfectly acquainted with all the Physical Knowledge pursuing at present in England; a frequent correspondent with Priestly, Magellan, and other England Philosophers, and a Man of Inventive Genius himself. I was however able to communicate to him some new Ideas which I pick'd up in my way, and which had not had time to reach him by way of England in a regular Course."[71] As Bentham hoped to launch a career in Russia working for the navy as an engineer, Guthrie provided an introduction to the secretary of the Admiralty and sponsored him for membership in the Free Economic Society, "here as it is a Society very much respected and I believe is very little if any expense; I shall certainly like it."[72]

Two weeks later, Bentham returned Guthrie's visit and was again impressed by Guthrie's knowledge. "I carried him some Books which were new to him as well as those he had lent me and brought back a few of his which were new to me; his House is filled with Subjects of natural Phillosophy. His Rooms were hung round all sorts chemicals in particular; He seems to have a compleat apparatus for Experiments in Airs; I shall probably get some Tables from him as will he perhaps one or two from me."[73] Later that week, the British envoy extraordinary presented Bentham to Catherine the Great and then followed that presentation with an introduction to Peter Simon Pallas at the Academy of Sciences.[74] These introductions facilitated Bentham's employment in the Admiralty, where he worked to improve the strength of timber used in shipbuilding. Within a year, the College of Manufacturing would hire him to inspect all mining operations throughout Siberia.

Men like Samuel Bentham justified the faith the Russian government placed in them. On his Siberian odyssey, he not only managed his assigned task but also gathered evidence to respond to Russia's critics. When traveling between Ekaterinburg and Nizhnii Tagil, for example, he noted: "The land about here is by no means unfertile, whatever the Abbé Chappe may say to the contrary. I saw yesterday some very promising crops of Corn, and all the ground which I saw cleared of wood produces something: when nothing is sown, there comes up a fine thick high grass."[75] Bentham sent this comment to his well-connected brother Jeremy in London in June 1781. Bentham was both familiar with the Chappe d'Auteroche's infamous text and dismissive of its claims upon his arrival in Siberia. His observations were relevant not only to his employer, the College of Manufacturing, and the British residing in St. Petersburg, like Guthrie, but also among members of the Royal Society in London. This combination of personal and professional networks continued to provide benefits for the empire's reputation.

The personal networks operating in St. Petersburg remained as small as ever, placing trusted men into key positions. Guthrie not only attempted to influence the view of Russia's management of its empire in British publications but also facilitated the employment of other British men into elite positions, not unlike how Peter the Great's physician, Robert Areskine, had done at the start of the century. Without doubt, the plague's arrival in Moscow in 1771 was a setback for Russia's international reputation as an innovator for health, but it quickly returned to business as usual. The state built new hospitals, hired more specialists, and promoted new therapies to redress its disease burden. It supported an active intervention to improve imperial health.

These ongoing improvements did not mean the Russian Empire had resolved all its health and population concerns. A small outbreak of the plague in the fall of 1780 once again raised an alarm. The British envoy extraordinary wrote to the foreign secretary in London, "Though it is kept here the most profound Secret, I can assure your Lordship that the Plague has broke out at a small Town formerly called Oel-Ecatherinskoy, situated in that Part of the Empire called Non-Russian on the River Bog, where the Frontiers of these Dominions of Moldavia, and of Poland, join." Although the envoy had concerns of exposure to the "dreadful Distemper," he confidently concluded, "the Coldness of the Winter will prevent its extending itself Northward."[76] As the plague did not become a widespread epidemic in 1781, his prediction was accurate, even if his reasoning was flawed. In fact, the absence of any further mention of the outbreak is a testament to the Russian government's successes since the devasting outbreak of 1771.

The state's employees in the Academy of Sciences and the College of Medicine worked to alter the criticism by highlighting their successes or even, as Guthrie did, Russia's peasants' ability to thrive in their extreme environment. In 1781, Catherine the Great invited Thomas Dimsdale to return to St. Petersburg, this time to inoculate her grandsons, the future tsar Aleksandr and his brother Konstantin. This posed another opportunity to draw attention to the medical interventions ongoing in the empire. Perhaps unsurprisingly, the event was anxiously watched by the British ambassador, as Britain's reputation was linked to Dimsdale's public role.[77] The princes were inoculated the last week of August at the palace: "There is as yet no appearance of the Distemper, but from their sound constitution, and very fine Season, there is little doubt of their doing perfectly well."[78] By the middle of September, both were recovered, though the court remained riveted by their mother's concern. As the ambassador noted, "The Young Great Dukes are now perfectly recovered of the Small Pox; The Eldest has had a very full distemper, and alarmed a good deal of the maternal affection of the Great Dutchess; the Other had a very slight Eruption."[79] The celebration for the success of the operation was highly public and ended with another award for Dimsdale, who "received from Her Imperial Majesty a gratification of ten thousand Pounds Sterling, two thousand pounds Sterling for his Journey backwards and forwards, and His Lady a diamond Ring of near One Thousand Pounds value."[80] At a time of diplomatic tensions between Britain and Russia from Britain's ongoing Atlantic wars during the American Revolution, Dimsdale's successful procedure and public acknowledgment would certainly have been a relief for Britain's diplomats. Following the setbacks to Russia's reputation from the outbreak of the plague and the equivocal evidence from Pallas's and Georgi's expedition, Dimsdale's success only highlighted the government's commitment to defeating smallpox, which, even in 1781, was still quite progressive compared with most European countries. There were undoubted benefits for both Russia's and Britain's reputations.

The empire's health care steadily improved from the investment in public interventions, but everyone remained aware of the dangers of Russia's climate. Visitors to the empire could easily observe both positive interventions and the intemperate climate on a single trip. Dimsdale's wife, Elizabeth, who accompanied him to Russian on the 1781 journey, did exactly that. In her diary, Elizabeth carefully noted the progress of her husband's latest patients, Aleksandr and Konstantin, with admiration for the treatment and concern at all levels of the palace. She also included some concerning observations about the climate. "It was during the Months of December, January and February, usually from 8 to 15 or 20 degrees below 0 that is from 40 to 52 degrees below the freezing Point: tho commonly in the course of Winter, it is for a Week or ten days some degrees lower." It was sufficiently cold, that it would be "difficult for an Inhabitant of our temperate Climate, to have any Idea of a cold so great." To Elizabeth, the dangers were obvious, as

"Drivers who sit on their loaded Carriages, are sometimes found frozen to death in that Position" at such temperatures. Even worse, "it is not unfrequent in the course of a Winter that some poor wretches getting drunk with Spirituous Liquors, fall down the road side, and perish before any one finds them."[81] Note that Elizabeth was only in Russia during the summer, so her knowledge of cold came from a particular source, her traveling companion, John Glen King. King's publication on climate may have argued that Russia's peasants could survive and thrive in these conditions, and yet Elizabeth's understanding of Russia from King, as recorded in her diary, suggested the opposite. King's publication was part of the public discussion about Russia's climate, but Elizabeth's diary revealed how difficult it was to shift the everyday experience of living in Russia, even for its most vocal advocates.

Chapter 6

Analyzing Catarrh, Overcoming Climate

Catherine's long reign alternated between positive health interventions and pandemic disasters. In the early years, a focus on gynecology and obstetrics, which were necessary for improving the birth rate, led to new specialists arriving. An expanded translation and publication program made information more accessible to the medical community. The triumph of the inoculation program begun by Thomas Dimsdale achieved international recognition. But the positive turn was unfortunately quick. The bubonic plague arrived in 1771, and, even if Russian practitioners developed a new fumigating powder to prevent transmission of which they were quite proud, it failed to make a deep impact outside of the country. After all, the expectation had been that Russia could provide solutions for cold diseases, such as scurvy, and not hot ones, such as the plague.

Evolving ideas about medicine, particularly disease transmission, posed another challenge for Russia's physicians. By the last quarter of the eighteenth century, if not earlier, the role of climate as a factor in the spread of diseases was being reevaluated. Some physicians advocated that particulate matter in the air was the key to disease transmission, in other words, that the miasma in the air was the issue, not the temperature or humidity. Others believed more strongly than ever that epidemic diseases must be transmitted from person to person, even if they were not certain what the specific vector was, as it could be called a contagion, germ, virus, or poison, depending on the author. Others yet still adhered to the role of climate and the danger of putrefaction in cold climates. For those physicians, the Russian Empire served as an important laboratory for observing illnesses with its extremely cold temperatures. The more the other positions held sway among physicians, however, the less valuable physicians in Russia became.

Reflecting the shift away from the value of Russia's physicians, the new imperial expeditions at the end of the century was guided less by scientific curiosity and more specifically by geopolitical concerns. The Second Kamchatka Expedition was a joint enterprise of the Academy of Sciences and the Admiralty, but that partnership was not guiding Joseph Billings's mission into the North Pacific in 1785 nor Russia's first circumnavigation under the direction of Adam Johann Ritter von Krusenstern in 1803. Physicians and naturalists still traveled with these expeditions, making observations about imperial subjects, their lifestyles, their overall health, and the disease burden. In many ways, narratives from the Billings and Krusenstern missions resemble those from the Second Kamchatka Expedition. Documenting the lack of improvements for the health of the empire, however, was hardly a resounding achievement at this moment. Part of the problem may have been how these narratives still linked the climate and health, relying on it as the reason why the population of the North Pacific region remained small. By the beginning of the nineteenth century, this was no longer a persuasive argument for most physicians, including those on the expeditions. Medical ideas had evolved beyond the sorts of information these expeditions produced.

Russia's Catarrh?

In 1782, the pandemic disease that overran Europe became known as the Russian catarrh. A catarrh was a cold disease, so its emergence from the coldest country seemed plausible. Ultimately, however, this incident revealed how the expectation of Europe's physicians increasingly differed from those practicing in Russia. Recording the outbreak served as a case study for ongoing debates about disease transmission. Labeling it a "Russian" catarrh served a second interest: What did the empire signify in Europe in the 1780s? Was Russia an unhealthy space that produced dangerous illnesses, or were Russia's subjects the first victims of an unavoidable pandemic?

Understanding catarrh was not a new problem in 1782. Catarrh pandemics were frequent in the eighteenth century, with the most recent emerging in 1775. Eighteen-century catarrh was not the same disease as the twentieth-first-century catarrh, though both involved the lungs. Dr. William Cullen, a professor at University of Edinburgh, wrote an updated nosological guide to diseases in Latin in 1769, which remained popular enough to be translated into English by the end of the century. According to Cullen, catarrhs belonged to the order Profluvia, a large category of diseases featuring fevers with "increased excretions not naturally bloody." Catarrhs were "often contagious; [with] encreased excretion of mucus, from the glands of the membrane of the nose, fauces, or bronchia, at least an effort at such excretion." The category "Catarrhus" included not only a variety of catarrhs but also coryza, rheumatism, and tussis. Cullen further divided catarrhs into two categories, "Catarrh from cold" and "Catarrh from contagion." The contagious category was marked as "epidemic" (either "Catarrhus epidemicus" or "Rheuma epidemicum"), whereas the cold versions were simply "Catarrrhus benignus" or "Coryza catarrhalis," among others.[1] A physician trained in Edinburgh before the 1775 or 1782 outbreak would have understood that a common catarrh was what we would call a cold, but epidemic catarrh was a contagious disease marked by a fever.[2] Italian physicians, by comparison, called epidemic catarrh an influenza, but most British physicians did not use that name until after 1782.[3]

When the 1782 catarrh arrived in Europe, physicians logically considered their experiences with the 1775 outbreak. In its wake, several physicians published their analysis of the disease, including a fellow of the Royal Society of London, Dr. John Mudge, in his *Radical and Expeditious Cure for a Recent Catarrhous Cough* (1779). He employed a nosological approach to the disease, placing epidemic catarrh among other conditions involving the lungs. He considered any disease of the lungs as a type of cold, which spanned a range from a cough to a fever, or even spitting blood; modern physicians might identify these as colds, influenza, and tuberculosis. Putrefaction was the primary cause of Mudge's broad category of colds. He explained that "the disorder we commonly call a Cold is generally supposed to be produced from a sudden check of perspiration, by the action of cold upon the surface of the body or the lungs." This could produce multiple symptoms, because "any sudden suppression or interruption of any excretion which is necessary to a sound state of the constitution, must be productive of mischief." If putrefaction of the humors was the precipitate cause, then Mudge was certain the climate was the underlying culprit, particularly in Britain. He suggested: "The sudden, and sometimes severe, changes of weather to which this climate is subject, are perhaps the most unhappy circumstances attending our situation; and the pernicious effects of them upon the human constitution are so frequently experienced, that diseases of the breast may be truly considered as endemical among the inhabitants of this island."[4]

Before the 1782 Russian catarrh, physicians had not agreed on the cause of a catarrh, nor was the term particularly stable as it could be applied to what modern physicians recognize as a wide range of diseases. Mudge believed catarrhs resulted from a cold climate causing putrefaction, but Cullen argued epidemic catarrh (influenza) was contagious, moving from person to person. The opportunity created by 1782 was to gather further evidence to reach an agreement on the primary cause.

One of the earliest mentions of the disease that became the 1782 pandemic was made by Samuel Bentham, during his inspection of Siberia's mines. As many travelers to Siberia would do, he traveled once the rivers were frozen to benefit from the ease of moving along icy rivers. He departed from St. Petersburg and arrived in Perm in October 1781. In a letter sent from Perm to his brother Jeremy in London, he mentioned he kept "as exact a journal as possible, of what passes." He intended to stay in Perm for "a week, or perhaps a fortnight longer." Although most of the letter described his investigation of local minerals and his aspirations for Siberian discoveries, completing this letter from Perm was delayed by "a cold in my head."[5] In his journal, he noted that he fell ill of "influenza" a week after this first letter on November 5 and suffered from symptoms for the following two days, before departing Perm on November 8.[6] He neither mentioned in any subsequent letter to Jeremy suffering from either influenza or a catarrh, nor did he note in his journal his cold of the last week of October. A later account would suggest the catarrh pandemic began in Siberia in the fall of 1781 and arrived in St. Petersburg the final week of December before spreading across Europe during the spring of 1782. The timing of Samuel Bentham's illness(es) would fit within this time frame, possibly making his influenza note the first written account of the future pandemic.

When the disease arrived in St. Petersburg, it was recognized as either an epidemic catarrh or influenza, depending on the author. James Harris, the first Earl of Malmesbury, was Britain's envoy extraordinary in Russia from 1777 to 1783. His regular dispatches to the British secretary of state for the Northern Department provide a detailed account of the outbreak. During the last week of December 1781, Harris mentioned that "The Cold still continues at 25 degrees & it is by far the severest winter I recollect to have felt."[7] Two weeks later, Harris observed "mild and damp Air which has prevailed here for these last eight or ten days has produced an almost universal Illness, similar to that which some years ago was called in London the *Influenza*, & in Paris *la Grippe*. I am the only one of the Corps diplomatique who has escaped it; It has affected Her Imperial Majesty in a slight degree, but I have the satisfaction to learn that She is to day intirely free from it." To Harris, the extreme cold of December followed by the unseasonable warmth of January resulted in this widespread outbreak. He was confident a return to cold weather would resolve the situation: "A few degrees of Frost which now seems probable, will soon restore health to every body." However, "I am satisfied that the Illness of the Empress and Prince Potemkin is not solely caused by the epidemical Air. Ill Humour and Dissatisfaction pervade the whole Palace and in these Moments all Business, however essential, is absolutely neglected."[8]

A week later, the situation had begun to improve. As Harris noted: "The universal Cold and Cough which has prevailed for these last ten days, now begin to diminish." As more news reached St. Petersburg, Harris now knew "it had been as General at Moscow as here." Harris was never concerned about the illness nor its effect on the public, but rather how it "occasioned an entire Suspension of Business and is the Cause why my letters have, these last two or three posts, been so uncommonly short and void of Matter."[9] As the cold weather continued in February, symptoms continued to abate. Harris wrote: "The weather has been again uncommonly severe; the Thermometer the night before last was at 30 degrees below the freezing point, and has never been less than 20 [degrees] since Monday. The Epidemical distemper diminishes; its Effects have been felt in every part of this neighbourhood, and I understand it has reached Courland and Polish Prussia."[10] Although Harris was not a physician, his letters provided an accurate account of the timing of the disease's arrival, its movement beyond Russia, and the common belief of the connection between the climate and the illness.

During the late winter and early spring of 1782, the illness traversed the Baltic region, arriving in Britain in May, and then returning to the Continent in the summer. Multiple physicians kept detailed notes on the pandemic. By the end of 1782, numerous publications on the pandemic began to circulate throughout Europe to contribute to the debate. Dr. Johann Daniel Metzger, a professor of medicine at

University of Königsburg, published a lengthy tract detailing the arrival of the disease, its symptoms, and potential treatments, compiling the knowledge gained through his correspondence with at least eight other physicians in northern Germany and at least one merchant in St. Petersburg. On the origins of the disease, Metzger detailed that it was popularly known as "the Russian, or the Northern disease." It was accepted that the disease arrived on the southern shore of the Baltic Sea from St. Petersburg and then moved through German lands. On its arrival, Metzger noted most people believed it to be a "miasmatic epidemic" (*epidemischen Miasma*), because of the swift progress of the infection. This idea, that particulates in the air were responsible for disease transmission, was a third theory of the cause of disease. Metzger did not believe the disease was contagious nor linked to the weather. Metzger's Russian informant, one "Herr Kant," wrote that the disease had arrived in St. Petersburg from Tobol'sk in Siberia. Metzger mentioned, however, that one of the other Germans living in St. Petersburg had been informed that the disease did not originate in Tobol'sk, but rather among the Tatars in Astrakhan, which raised the possibility of Middle Eastern origins like the plague a decade earlier.[11]

By contrast, in a summary report produced by the medical faculty of the University of Paris in 1782, the weather was the primary cause of the pandemic. As the report noted, an "intermittent fever" was circulating during warm weather, but it "yielded easily to ordinary treatment." However, once the temperature "changed from hot to cold, the illness soon took on another character; the intermittent fever became continuous." This illness had several accompanying symptoms, but medical faculty agreed it was most appropriately considered a "catarrhal infection" or "the grippe," as it resembled the earlier outbreak in 1776.[12]

Metzger believed the catarrh pandemic was miasmatic in origin; the University of Paris believed the weather was to blame. Some physicians in Britain, Cullen among them, had already concluded that catarrhs were contagious, moving from person to person, not through the air as others argued. By 1784, when the Society for the Promotion of Medical Knowledge in London compiled its data on the outbreak from across Britain, it agreed that the catarrh must be contagious. The society's report was written by Dr. Edward Whitaker Gray. Before joining the society, Gray had become the keeper of the natural history collection for the British Museum in 1778, and he had been elected a fellow of the Royal Society in 1779. He published in both *Philosophical Transactions* for the Royal Society and two catalogs of the collections at the British

Museum. All these roles positioned Gray in the middle of knowledge networks spanning Europe in the late eighteenth century. As a result, his article on the pandemic for the Society for the Promotion of Medical Knowledge circulated in Europe, including a German translation in 1785, as part of *Medicinische Beyträge* (Gottingen).[13]

Gray produced a detailed assessment of the pandemic outbreak, drawing on multiple British correspondents who were cited throughout as well as references to Metzger's and the University of Paris's publications. Gray was straightforward in his conclusion that the disease was an epidemic catarrh, as defined in Cullen's nosological study. According to Gray, "Very little authentic information has been procured, respecting the history of the disorder, before the time of its appearance in London; all that can upon good authority be related, is, that it prevailed at Moscow, in the months of December 1781, and January 1782, and at St. Petersburgh, in February 1782: it was traced from Tobolski, to which place it was supposed to have been brought from China."[14] It appears that Metzger was Gray's source for the early outbreak, as Metzger was the only European account to mention Tobol'sk as a site of infection. Metzger was clear, however, that Astrakhan and its Tatars were the likely source of the illness in Russia, not China. Russian authorities had long believed Astrakhan was a vulnerable spot for new diseases to arrive from the Middle East and South Asia, adopting a quarantine system for the city as early as the 1730s.[15] It is possible that Gray simply failed to understand the significance of Astrakhan as a potential origin site, or he was predisposed to assume a Chinese origin for the new illness.

Once the disease left St. Petersburg, according to Gray, its path followed that of the one established in the earlier accounts. The catarrh arrived in "Denmark the latter end of April, or the beginning of May; and many people were said to have died to it at Copenhagen, before the 11th of May. It is not easy to determine with precision, the time of its first appearance in London; that it was here the second week in May, seems very certain." It then traveled back across the Continent and into the Mediterranean region from France in June to Italy in July and to Portugal and Spain in August and September. Gray reported a similar illness had been observed in "different parts of the East Indies" in "the months of October and November 1781," but it was not clear if it was the same illness.[16]

The list of symptoms was exhaustive, including typical influenza markers such as fevers and chills, coughing, inflammation, and pains. Some symptoms were more atypical, including "bleeding from the nose; spitting of blood; loss of smell or taste; nausea; flatulence." In general, Gray rarely passed judgment on the long list, finally concluding the "others were remarked as evident signs of a tendency to putrefaction; and in one case, the disease seems to have put on the form of a nervous disorder." As Gray admitted, "Various, and even contradictory, as the forementioned symptoms appear, their right to be considered as belonging to the influenza, or at least as having been caused by it, will, perhaps, be admitted, when it is observed, that this disorder (as has been remarked of former epidemics) excited, and become complicated with, those complaints to which the persons affected were, from local situation, or constitution, most predisposed."[17]

Following Gray's reviews of the broad range of symptoms with a detailed account of all the various treatments attempted, the outstanding issue to be resolved was to identify the disease and explain its spread. Gray summarized the debate: "Some physicians thought it arose solely from the state of the weather; in other words, that it was a common catarrh, occasioned, as that complaint frequently is, by changes in the sensible qualities of the atmosphere, such as the increase of cold, or moisture; . . . Others, admitted its cause to be a particular and specific contagion, totally different from, and independent, of the sensible qualities of the atmosphere, yet thought that cause was conveyed by, and resided in the air." Gray's correspondents, however, reached a different assessment: "that the influenza was contagious, in the common acceptation of that word, that it is to say, that it was conveyed and propagated by the contact, or at least by the sufficiently near approach, of an infected person." Gray's assessment systematically rejected any connection of this catarrh to the weather, which was the neo-Hippocratic theory. Gray offered a simple rebuttal to this theory: "Another remarkable fact remains to be taken notice of; which, though it is not mentioned as an argument of very great weight, certainly merits some consideration. The influenza prevailed in Russia in the months of December, January, and February, and in Italy and Spain in the months of July, August, and September, consequently its cause must have been capable of resisting almost the two extremes of European heat and cold; a degree of permanence difficult to be conceived, if we suppose that cause to have resided in the air."[18] In other words, the absence of evidence to support the climatic or miasmatic positions, coupled with the ability to trace the geography of a transmission vector from Russia to Britain and then back to the Continent, left Gray, and the Society for the Promotion of Medical Knowledge, with one conclusion: This disease was contagious.

At the same time, Russia's physicians notably had been missing from the published accounts on Russia's catarrh. Although European physicians debated its origins, they seemingly had little interest in what those living in Russia experienced, beyond Metzger's correspondence with a German merchant in St. Petersburg. In 1791, a decade after the outbreak, the first account of a physician who had worked in Russia was published. This account was written by Charles de Mertens, who once again relied on his Russian career from 1767 to 1773 to provide his insight. Unlike his short text in *Philosophical Transactions* on scurvy, this 1791 publication was a two-volume analysis about diseases in general, drawing on his career in the Russian Empire for evidence. It was written in Latin and published in Pavia, while he was teaching in Vienna.[19] Because he published his account a decade after leaving Russia, the connection to his time in Moscow may not have been immediately obvious to some readers. Even with those caveats, it remains the only narrative published in the eighteenth century by a physician who had practiced in Russia.

Mertens's chapter on "The Catarrhal Fever" of 1782 was subtitled "The Russian Disease [*morbus Russicus*], the Grippe, called Influenza." Like most accounts of the disease, he began with a description of the unusual weather that preceded the outbreak: A "scorching summer in 1781, when the heat and rain continued for three months" was followed by "a very hot and dry season" the following autumn. From correspondents in Russia, he received news from St. Petersburg in January 1782 that the temperature jumped "30 degrees in the space of a day. On the same day they reported that about 40,000 men had been seized with a catarrhal fever, and that scarcely a sufficient number of healthy men had been found for the vigil among the numerous troops; that the said fever had promiscuously attacked the nobles' servants, and the servants in the court, but few succumbed to the disease, which only lasted for a few days, leaving many of them weak and infirm." Following the arrival of disease in St. Petersburg, it traveled to "Sweden, Denmark, and the circle of Lower and Upper Saxony were visited by a fever epidemic, which many, because of its place of origin, called the Russian disease, but the English called influenza."[20] Several points differed in the origin of the illness in Mertens's view. It began in St. Petersburg, not Siberia or China, and the precipitating cause was clearly the weather, which was the neo-Hippocratic position.

Mertens did not offer a time frame or explanation how the disease moved from St. Petersburg to Moscow. He did provide, however, a list of symptoms recorded in patients who were treated in the city. Patients "feel tired and horrified, and are soon seized with a cold, with cough, coryza, pain in the head and chest, somewhat difficult breathing, and stiffness. These symptoms became worse on the second day with the subsequent fever. . . . They feel rheumatic pains in the neck, shoulders, and chest; but they have a constant pain under the upper part of the sternum, in the lungs, throat, and increased coughing. In conclusion, "The symptoms observed in most people in our country indicated that this epidemic disease was a true rheumatic or catarrhal fever, more or less, but, in general, only slightly inflammatory; the fever of this slight inflammation was chiefly found in the internal and external parts of the chest."[21] Although Mertens's argument on the origin of the disease differed from most writing in Europe at the time, his list of symptoms neatly matches the other accounts circulating across the Continent. It may be that his advocacy for the climatic origins a decade after a consensus emerged that it was in fact contagious, allowed his observations to be dismissed as irrelevant, or, at least, uninformed.

The documentation produced in the wake of the catarrh pandemic of 1781–1782 reflected firsthand observations. There was broad consensus on the symptoms of the disease and acceptance that it was an epidemic catarrh, as that disease was understood by the nosologists. At the same time, some issues were unresolved. The origin of the disease remained debated, as some in Britain argued for at least Siberian, if not Chinese origins, some physicians in Germany like Metzger pointed to Astrakhan and the Middle East, whereas Mertens believed it began in St. Petersburg. The evidence of men such as Samuel Bentham who diagnosed himself with influenza a month before the disease arrived in St. Petersburg would challenge those who believed in its origin in Petersburg, but that evidence lived in his personal notebook, not in the published accounts. The method of transmission remained debated, as advocates for climatic, miasmatic, and contagionist views all weighed in. The British establishment primarily backed contagionism, but those practicing on the Continent were less persuaded. Knowing that medical evidence failed to persuade the public that the pandemic was not a Russian catarrh, it is plausible that contagionism was not as popular with the broad public as it was with Britain's physicians.

The catarrh pandemic reveals the difficulty of achieving consensus in the medical community at the end of the eighteenth century. With the prominent roles for Edinburgh-trained physicians in Russia, it may not be a surprise that the British medical community advocated for a Chinese origin for the recent pandemic. After all, that shifted responsibility for the European pandemic from Russia and its Anglo-Russian trade network. In fact, it was only the physician who left his position in Russia who remained committed to a Russian origin. This debate, however, uncovered a serious issue. Whereas Russian expertise on scurvy was once sought as particularly valuable, no one in Europe thought physicians in Russia might have knowledge of the so-called Russian catarrh. Part of the reason for this shifting view was the evolution of disease theory in the eighteenth century. For those who still believed that climate was a primary factor in health, Russia offered a unique opportunity to observe the consequences of cold temperatures on bodies. For those who believed that disease was contagious or miasmatic, Russia was no longer exceptional. The causes of disease were far more immediate than the climate or geography.

Those diplomats who were involved in recording the events were not particularly helpful. James Harris, whose letters to the British government detailed the outbreak in the winter of 1781 and 1782, easily dismissed its consequences by the summer once it departed Britain for the Continent. In fact, Harris's primary concern shifted to his health and the persistence of Russia's unhealthy climate. In September 1782, he wrote to the foreign secretary, "My distemper is an annual or rather continual tribute I pay to this climat from the Autumnal to the Vernal Equinox – it never begun so violently as now and I cannot yet see where it will end." Harris argued that only one outcome was possible: "[If] I stay here much longer that it will so far break my Constitution as to make the Remainder of my life of a Period of Infirmity. I have every year felt more & more the bad effect of this Air, & the Strictist Attention to every thing which contributes to Health has not been able to preserve me from its baneful Influence."[22] His complaints resembled so many of his predecessors in St. Petersburg, and his goal, like theirs, was to be recalled to Britain. In the face of an actual dangerous pandemic, Harris was steadfast; in the face of the regular fall weather, he simply crumbled. Russia's climate continued to break the spirit of its residents, who could now turn to former employees like Mertens for further proof of the dangers.

Resolving Climate

Disease theory moved away from emphasizing the role of climate; remarkably, however, the label of the Russian catarrh remained into the twentieth century, even as epidemic catarrh became known as influenza.[23] The popular, not medical, idea that Russia was a country where diseases emerged persisted. It is not a surprise, therefore, that those men still in Russia's employment actively defended Russia's healthy qualities. Physicians such as Matthew Guthrie continued to publish studies praising Russians' ability to manage their environment, and his fellow state employees offered new evidence about the empire's ability to manage its disease burden. Perhaps more helpfully, by the end of the eighteenth century, physicians were increasingly cynical about the connection of climate to health, which steadily eroded the long-held opinion of the Russian Empire as an unhealthy space.

In 1785, Guthrie published a pamphlet in St. Petersburg in French, *Nouvelles experiences pour servir à determiner le vrai point de congelation du mercure*, providing updated information on the academy's ongoing investigation of the freezing point of mercury.[24] Having conducted a series of experiments, Guthrie's conclusion was that Peter Simon Pallas's work in Siberia had been confirmed by his own work in St. Petersburg. Guthrie's conclusions were summarized in *Medical Commentaries* in Edinburgh the following year, which also added the contents of one of Guthrie's recent letters on the treatment of a young boy in St. Petersburg suffering from rabies. Guthrie first examined the patient, insisting on treatment with a "strong mercurial ointment" that was used on the bite wound for fourteen days. Then, against Guthrie's orders, the boy was treated with "Ormskirk medicine" as the "remedy looked specific in his native county, Derbyshire," which was used for five weeks, until he could once again no longer walk and suffered from fevers. Guthrie then stopped treatment with the Ormskirk remedy, and returned to the mercurial ointment, which led to a full recovery. Guthrie's conclusion was that the English remedy failed to work in Russia, whereas the extreme heat of the mercury treatment could succeed.[25]

Following his experiments with mercury, Guthrie returned to the primary challenge of Russia: scurvy. In a letter to *Medical Commentaries*, Guthrie noted that many physicians had discussed "the influence of hot climates on the human body, and its diseases; but few seem to have investigated the effects of cold," excepting, of course, his own work on the subject, and arguably neglecting Johann Amman, John Cook, and all of the academy's specialists. Following his earlier letter to *Philosophical Transactions*, Guthrie observed an "extraordinary" scurvy outbreak in St. Petersburg in 1785. "A crop of cabbage, cucumbers, carrots, turnips, &c. having failed that year" left the navy incapable of providing the necessary provisions for its sailors, resulting in record numbers of patients in Kronstadt. The naval hospital had attempted to treat its patients with a locally sourced supply of "berries deservedly reckoned highly anti-scorbutic," but it was discovered that while the berries might prevent scurvy, they did little to ease the symptoms of an active case. Guthrie recommended that the best course of action was "to thin the crowded scorbutic wards, where the foul air evidently retarded their cure" as berries alone had not been sufficient. Furthermore, they adjusted the heat in the wards to the "sweating point" along with a "a deluge of diluting fluids to bring moisture on the skin" as a method to solve the putrefaction that was the source of the scurvy.[26]

Guthrie's work remained pivotal for the Russian government to shed the negative image spread by its critics in terms of the long-term damage done by its unchecked diseases. For example, Jean-Baptiste Barthélemy de Lesseps was appointed as the vice consul in St. Petersburg for France in 1783. Two years later, he was assigned to the Pacific Expedition of Jean-François de Galaup, comte de Lapérouse, to serve as a Russian translator in the North Pacific. In 1787, the expedition left Lesseps in Kamchatka to return to Paris with copies of the expedition's findings from the Pacific. It would take more than a year for Lesseps to cross Eurasia to depart for France from St. Petersburg, but his journey informed his travel narrative about life in Kamchatka and Siberia. Similar to Jean-Baptiste Chappe d'Auteroche, he was not complimentary about Russia's management of its imperial peoples. He suggested that the Russians had introduced smallpox in Kamchatka only in 1767 or 1768, and it had already eliminated three-fourths of the population on the peninsula. In addition, he noted: "There is reason to suspect that the Kamtschadales are indebted to them [the Russians] in like manner for their knowledge of the venereal disease . . . This pestilence appears to be exotic, and its cure is as difficult as it is rare. They have recourse to various roots and to corrosive sublimate, which is attended in this country with its usual ruinous effects, and the more so, as being indiscreetly administered."[27] Although he believed venereal disease was rare in Kamchatka, it was further proof of the damage the Russians had caused across the empire. His argument had already been contradicted by Johann Gottlieb Georgi, but condemning Russia potentially outweighed accuracy.

In light of the ongoing criticism, Russia's naturalists still needed evidence of their mastery of the climate. Guthrie drew on the data recorded by the academy's long-term project to detail the climate for his final assessment, "A Dissertation on the Climate of Russia" (1790). He relied on the academy's previous fifteen years of weather and temperature records. Guthrie adopted the standard practice of the academy of dividing "the year into two seasons only, as in fact we have but two, properly speaking, *viz.* winter and summer, the one season running into the other, without leaving well defined intermediate periods." From the evidence and his personal experiences, Guthrie concluded that "winter certainly must take the lead, . . . both from its duration and consequences in this northern situation. The duration of winter is generally from the end of September to the beginning of May." Although winter may have dominated the year, "the air, though cold, is remarkably pure and elastic during our severe frost, so as to give a most surprising degree of spring and tone to the human frame."[28]

Guthrie's observations and the academy's climate data produced a positive assessment of the climate. "The severity of the frost" did not lead to suffering from the winter, "but the fact is just the reverse: for people in easy circumstances, who are not obliged to remain much out of doors, but drive, or even walk from one house to another, suffer less than in most countries." Following his earlier discussion of the weather, Guthrie reiterated that "the warm fur dress [keeps] the body so comfortable, that I am convinced less cold is felt (differences of dress considered) in driving through the streets of Petersburgh in our cold dry air, than through those of London or Edinburgh, during the cold moist weather that obtains there during a great part of the winter; especially as this state of the atmosphere in Britain is often accompanied by bleak winds, whilst the air in Russia, during our greatest cold, is generally serene and calm." Only those among Russia's elite and foreigners who refused to adopt the correct habits suffered from cold, "because neither the houses nor dress are calculated to keep it [cold] from constantly acting on the body."[29]

According to the academy's data, the coldest month was January, when the temperature averaged 24°F below 0°F, but the "mean cold for the six winter months, is, in the afternoon, equal to 27° Fahr. above 0." The coldest temperature recorded in the previous fifteen years was −62° Fahr, which could be "often felt." Although "the whole surface of the northern countries is covered with snow to a considerable depth, over which we drive in sledges, without distinguishing between land and water," the average precipitation in the six months of winter was only five inches. By comparison, the six months of summer averaged eleven inches of rain.[30] Guthrie reported the data from the Academy of Sciences for 1774 to 1789, but the sixteen inches of rain per year average he noted was well below the modern average rainfall of nearly twenty-five inches.[31] If the academy's data were reliable, then one reason for the cold dry air of St. Petersburg may not have been from the peculiarity of Russia's climate, but rather from a particularly dry era of its history. Therefore, Guthrie's conclusions about the connection between climate and health may be faulty not from the data but instead from the atypical nature of Russia's climate in the 1770s and 1780s.

The year after Guthrie published his final word on Russia's climate, Mertens's volumes on disease were published. The first part continued his analysis of various epidemics, including the 1782 catarrh as discussed earlier, but Mertens's experiences in Russia were included throughout the text. The other diseases included were exactly the ones a physician in Russia would discuss—scurvy, smallpox, and syphilis. The chapter on scurvy was a reprint of the article he published in 1778 in *Philosophical Transactions*, in which he argued that the Russian peasant diet with its reliance on fresh vegetables, particularly "onions, leeks, turnips, and peas" was far more important for their ability to avoid scurvy than the bania. Scurvy was common in Russian cities because the elite avoided this diet in favor of preserved foods with too much salt.[32] The three chapters on smallpox inoculation reiterated the benefits of the Suttonian Method as it was used in Russia, and discussed his subsequent practice in Vienna.

The chapter on syphilis, however, offered new information drawn from his Russian career. Syphilis was an "evil disease which shortens men's lives. . . . It afflicts men with various tortures and after a miserable life usually leads them to the grave at a slow pace; it suffocates them at the very source of future offspring." Mertens found the persistence of syphilis the most troubling, as there was no reason it "should still exist among the peoples of Europe, when we have a specific remedy against it." The remedy was a compound of mercury. He wrote: "While I lived in Moscow from 1767 to 1773, I did not hear of the people or inhabitants using it as a remedy; but foreign physicians did use it." Mertens believed this was a problem only for urban residents and the elite, as he had investigated how Siberians resolved the disease. According to the College of Medicine in St. Petersburg, some Siberians had developed their own cure, taking a "sublimate of mercury" followed by the bania, where they would spend one hour per day until the "symptoms disappeared."[33] Unlike so much of what had been written about Russia, Mertens believed that syphilis remained a problem in Russia's cities, but it had been resolved with a local solution in Siberia, despite the frequent comment of its occurrence.

In his discussion of the catarrh pandemic, Mertens was clear that Russia's extremely cold climate caused the disease. In his discussion of the endemic diseases, scurvy and syphilis, the climate may have posed a challenge for treatment, but Russian peasants and Siberians developed solutions to each. In both cases, he identified urban elites as the ones incapable of addressing these illnesses, even when remedies were available. He was not writing in response to Guthrie's dissertation, but Mertens's conclusion that the population had long since adapted to its climate was consistent with his former colleague's view.

Guthrie's and Mertens's assessments reflected a turn away from belief that the climate was a primary cause of ill health by the 1790s. They were not alone. William Tooke was a member of the Russian Academy of Sciences and the English translator for Georgi's description of the empire. Although he was not a physician, his work at the academy influenced his comprehensive depiction of the empire in 1799. It borrowed Georgi's categorization of the population of the empire, but Tooke was far more critical about the impact of the climate on physical bodies.[34]

Tooke acknowledged that some had argued that the cold "be the occasion of certain epidemical diseases," but he was not convinced it was the only cause. As he explained, "delicate persons, especially of the higher classes, colds, defluxions, rheums, and coughs, are common enough, not merely during the cold of winter, but also at other seasons of the year: the common people know but little of these complaints. These never feel any injury from currents of air, which we call draughts; although persons of the former description frequently take cold even when they have not stirred out of their warm apartments." Tooke further explained that even "sharp biting frosts" could be managed, "if people are but properly clad, and forbear to sit down, especially upon the banks of snow, which may often cost them their lives."[35] Although Tooke was dismissive of the probability that the temperature had an effect on the body, he retained a fully articulated belief in the effects of the humors on the body.

In his second volume, Tooke began his description of the peoples of the empire by mentioning that "the bodily state of the people is dependent on a thousand things; nature of the soil, climate, weather; way of life, dress, food; manners and usages, even political constitution and religion have a decisive influence on the strength, the durability, the health, in short, the whole physical character of mankind." Any educated person of the eighteenth century would recognize Tooke's list of influences as Galen's nonnaturals. To accept the influence of the nonnaturals was to accept the importance of "airs" on a body's health. Tooke explicitly stated, however, that a "great number of persons in all these parts attain to a very advanced old age," which was "one sure proof that in general the climate is not prejudicial to health."[36]

Tooke may not have been a physician, but his interest in including a discussion about climate and health reflects how important this idea had been over the previous century. As part of the medical establishment in Russia, Guthrie offered his dissertation as the final evaluation on the issue. His evidence proved that Russia was objectively cold, but he also concluded that this was not a challenge for the empire's population. Others outside of Russia, like Lesseps, might continue to comment on how the Russian government failed to redress the damage done by scurvy, smallpox, and syphilis, but Russia's physicians were far more confident that these diseases were sufficiently controlled, at least among the peasantry.

Pacific Expeditions

As was often the issue, the Russian Empire was not only confronted by disease outbreaks and foreign critics of its policies but also by geopolitical concerns. Britain was frequently the source of those challenges. The two empires might have been dependent on their economic relationship, but Britain's explorations of the North Pacific, led by Captain James Cook, threatened Russia's expansion into the region (figure 6.1). Each of Cook's voyages was reported in Russia, including his death during his third voyage in 1779. Britain's foreign secretary informed the envoy extraordinary, James Harris, of Cook's death in January 1780. In Britain, it was a matter of "universal concern" and a "publick Misfortune."[37] It is not clear if Russia's court would have shared the concern, but the outcome of the Cook's third voyage was to send copies of Cook's new navigation charts and maps for "the North East Coasts of the Empress of Russia's Dominions & the North West Coasts of America" to Russia as a gift for the court.[38] By April, Britain's new charts of the North Pacific, demonstrating that Russia's "dominions" in the Pacific existed only in Asia, and not in North America, were dispatched.[39] Russia's claims were intentionally being threatened.

The solution to this implied threat was for the Russian government to launch another major expedition. Its primary task was not to further describe the land and peoples of the North Pacific, although it would

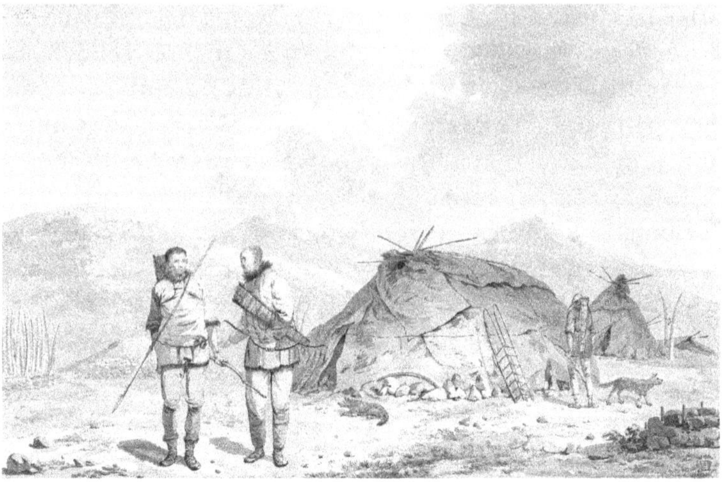

FIGURE 6.1. Captain Cook's third voyage not only mapped the North Pacific but also completed ethnographic studies in Eurasia, including this observation of the Chukchi on the Kamchatkan Peninsula. "Two Chukchi of the Chukotskiy Peninsula, Russia, in front of summer huts (yarangas)," in *Ninety Drawings, Some in Indian Ink, Some Coloured*, executed by J. Webber during the Third Voyage of Captain Cook (1776–1780). From the British Library Archive.

include naturalists, but rather to address the political concern of mapping the coastline as proof of Russia's possessions. In its response to Britain's challenge, the Russian government turned toward a British naval officer, Captain Joseph Billings, who had been the astronomer on the first Cook expedition. After that voyage, Billings had sought employment as a captain with the East India Company (EIC), offering them a proposal to expand their trade in the North Pacific. His plan was blocked by the Hudson's Bay Company, leading the EIC to deny Billings's request. Billings then took his proposal for his investigation of resources in the region, as well as new maps and navigation charts, to Russia.[40]

The Billings Expedition was another multiyear undertaking, beginning in 1785 and returning in 1795. He was given a Russian cocommander, Gavril Andreevich Sarychev, who had enlisted in the Russian Navy in 1781. The Englishman Martin Sauer was the official secretary of the expedition, and his account of the journey included records from Billings and many other participants, including its naturalists. One of those naturalists, Carl Heinrich Merck, would later write his own narrative. Merck was born in 1761 in Germany and received his medical degree at the University of Jena before entering Russian service.

Sarychev, who became an honorary member of the Academy of Sciences upon the expedition's conclusion, would also publish a narrative describing the events.[41]

As was the case for the Second Kamchatka or the Pallas Expedition, international interest in this latest effort was high. George Macartney, the British ambassador extraordinary sent to Russia to finalize a new trade treaty in 1786, included an update on the expedition's progress to the foreign secretary in London: "The following is the state of the expedition to those Countries under the Command of Captain Billings. He set out in June 1785. He was to go first to Jakutsk, then to Ochetskoi, then to the River Kolyma, to go down to the Mouth of it, and as far to the Eastward as the Season will permit. In the meanwhile the Ships are getting ready at Ochetskoi, As soon as he can in the Year 1787, he is to sail from Ochetskoi to the harbour of St. Peter and St. Paul."[42] Despite this interest, or perhaps because of it, the findings of the expedition were kept private in Russia until the nineteenth century. Sauer would leave Russia and publish his report from Britain in 1802, seven years after the expedition's end, and Sarychev's report would follow from Russia after that.

The absence of an official report immediately following the expedition's return provided Billings with an opportunity to exploit his information to further his career. He provided the EIC an update on his travels and Russia's interest in the North Pacific. It is perfectly in keeping with the history of Russia's naturalists to exploit their discoveries for their own gains, but Billings's actions are notable as he was also involved in delaying Sauer's publication on behalf of the Academy of Sciences.[43] Billings provided the East India Company's secretary the details of his instructions: "The Empress" outlined a series of tasks for his expedition. The first were cartographic: "1st to measure by a chain, where it was practicable, the distances between several places which the Empress names in Her Instruction. . . . 2) To determine the latitude and longitude of places with the utmost exactness. . . . 3) To make plans, drawings, views, &c." The second category was designed simply to continue the typical scientific work of the expedition, "To collect specimens of Mineralogy & Natural History." The third category was intended to investigate the condition of the empire's American subjects: "To enquire into the abuses, and acts of cruelty and oppression, committed by the Russians in those distant parts, on the original inhabitants. The account he gives of the conduct of the Russians towards those poor defenseless people is so shocking, that it appears almost incredible, but horrid as it is, it is corroborated by the testimony of the Russians themselves." The final category was geopolitical, as Catherine's government was invested in its control of the North Pacific. The expedition should "proceed down the Coast of America as far as Mount Elias. 7) To find a port proper for established an Admiralty for building and repairing ships, both for War and commerce; 8) To discover whether the sea is at anytime open between the Continents of Asia and America, so as to permit a vessel to said round to the West. 9) To go to the utmost northern extreme of Chutkoi (or Tschutka). 10) To determine, as near as possible, the number of Inhabitants in every place he went to. 11) To make an exact survey of the Coast of America, and particularly to give a correct account of the Harbours." Although the directions provided a detailed explanation of the goals of the expedition, the EIC must have been relieved to hear that Billings "made no discoveries of new lands or islands," even though he "has gained a more perfect knowledge of all those parts, of which before their notions were very vague and erroneous." Some of this new information concerned the climate. Billings confirmed that "the Ice never thaws between Cape Chalatskoi and the American Continent," although "the water is open in summer through the Straits of Behring almost to the point of Chalatskoi."

Beyond geography, Billings's assessment was not complimentary to Russia's management of its possessions. He found Kamchatka to be "very miserable, and there are only 700 souls remaining of the aborigines, the rest having been extirpated by the Russians." It was no better on the American side. Billings wrote: "The Russians are depopulating very fast both their own Islands and the Continent of America. In the islands they drive the inhabitant out into the woods to hunt for furs in the most severe weather, where great numbers of them perish. They plunder them of this property and provisions, so that whole families frequently perish by famine. They consistently turn them ill, and often kill them. When the Russians return to their own country they carry of as many women and children as they can conduct, and make slaves of them for their own use, or sell them." Billings even provided evidence that some of Russia's territorial claims were illegitimate. He confirmed that "the Island which a Russian trade, and an adventurer in those parts pretended to discover," was in fact "the island of Kirtak (or rather Kistak) discovered by Captain Cook."[44] If Billings had been dispatched by the Russian government to produce new maps to confirm their possession in the North Pacific, it seems doubtful it would have been pleased with his confirmation of a British discovery of a contested island.

Billings's information provided to the EIC was no worse than Chappe d'Auteroche's view of Russia's effect on Siberia's population. One difference was that Billings provided this information privately as he sought employment, rather than in print. Billings followed the example of his fellow countrymen, particularly the diplomats, who often criticized Russia in their dispatches to London but who wisely kept these complaints private to avoid the tsar's irritation.

If Billings was so critical of Russia's mismanagement in private, the need for the government to present the expedition as a great achievement was only that much more difficult. Certainly having Sauer depart Russian service, and the empire, before publishing his notes from the expedition added to the concern about how the information could be used. At the same time, Sauer's comments would hardly have been surprising to anyone familiar with the publications of the previous expeditions. In Okhotsk, he lamented the climate: "The air is unwholesome in the extreme, as fogs, mists, and chilling winds, constantly prevail, which so much affect the products of the earth, that nothing grows within five versts of the sea." The air contributed to the ill health of the inhabitants, who suffered from poor habits as well as geography. Sauer added: "The scurvy rages here with great violence, owing, perhaps, as much to want of attention and cleanliness in the inhabitants, as to the climate."[45]

Sauer's descriptions of the local populations borrowed from his predecessors and also noted the damage still done by endemic diseases. The Iakuts, for example, "are a healthy and hardy race, bear the extremes of heat and cold to an astonishing degree, and travel in the severest frosts on horseback, frequently suffering much from hunger; they are, however, subject to rheumatic pains, boils, the itch, and fore eyes; and great numbers were carried off in 1758 and 1774 by the small-pox and measles."[46] By the time Sauer published, men like Guthrie and Mertens had argued that the Russian population, especially in Siberia, were successfully adapted to their climate. Sauer's comments offered a rebuttal of those comments with a reminder of the devastation of smallpox and the mention of rheumatism, which Guthrie had included in his discussion of Siberian treatments in his 1777 article in *Medical and Philosophical Commentaries*.[47]

Unlike Pallas and Georgi's expedition, Billings and Sauer traversed the North Pacific, adding Indigenous Alaskans to their description of the peoples of the empire. Although Sauer may have drawn on the preexisting descriptions of the Siberian population, he was breaking new ground for the Indigenous communities of North America. Sauer's portrayals relied on similar language and ideas, but frequently sketched contradictory types of bodies. In Carl Linnaeus's taxonomy, Native Americans were one of the four categories of humankind, separated from Europeans and Asians.[48] The evidence from the Billings Expedition, however, seemed to describe them as part of a broader mixed category that included many of the peoples of Siberia. On Kodiak Island, for example, Sauer described the male Kodiaks of having two occupations: "The first character, is the athletic and skillful warrior; the second, the fleet and expert hunter; the former enjoys his prisoners and the booty of the enemy; the latter has his wives, labourers, and slaves by purchase, and the ability that he possesses to maintain them." His description of active, athletic men suggested hot body types, which was potentially surprising considering the location. Kodiak women confirmed this diagnosis, as "the most favoured of women is she who has the greatest number of children." Fertility was always associated with heat, not cold. The children of Kodiak, however, raised some questions for Sauer, but he blamed the outcome on their childrearing practices: "The women seem very fond of their offspring; dreading the effects of war, and the dangers of the chase; some of them bring up their males in a very effeminate manner, and are happy to see them taken by the chiefs, to gratify their unnatural desires. Such youths are dressed like women, and taught all their domestic duties."[49] The Kodiak population were different from those people living in Kamchatka, but Sauer's interest in their physical activities and procreative habits fits neatly into the types of information Russia's naturalists had been recording for decades.

Sauer's choice to first publish his narrative in London in English, instead of through the Russian Academy, raised questions about his intentions. Certainly, he frustrated Billings's interest in furtively passing information to the EIC about Russia's interest in the Pacific by making the expedition's work public. Sauer's account was also followed by the official accounts endorsed by the academy that were published by Sarychev and later Merck. Both accounts did more to confirm Sauer's report than to raise questions of its validity. Sarychev, for example, described Okhotsk in similar terms: "The weather is cold and damp the greater part of the year, and not unfrequently so in that season when heat is indispensable for bringing the corn to maturity. For this reason, the vegetables and garden fruits are far inferior to those in other places lying nearer to the north pole, where, as in Archangel for example, they have a better climate."[50] Sauer may have said "nothing" grew in Okhotsk, but Sarychev was hardly complimentary.

Merck's account, like Sauer's, offered ample examples of the widespread disease burden among Russia's subjects. On Kodiak, for example, he noted: "External infections, also in the face, sore throat, abscesses in throat and nose, pain in the bones, deterioration of the bone which causes their bones to break. Syphilis is present from long ago." Although the pervasive diseases suggested an unhealthy populace, "nevertheless, they do grow old so that they can hardly walk under the burden of years."[51] Merck may not have published to support Sauer's assessment, but his physical descriptions only confirmed Sauer's belief in the hot qualities of the Kodiaks.

Aside from the common ideas shared among the three men in terms of geography, climate, and population, once scurvy overtook the expedition's crew in the fall of 1790, each narrative focused on uncovering potential scurvy treatments. Both Sauer and Merck quoted one of the crew's surgeons, a Mr. Roebeck: "It was only towards the end of the voyage, when our bread was out, and we were reduced to a short allowance of water, that the scurvy made its appearance. At this time pease and grits boiled to a thick consistency in a small quantity of water, and buttered, were substituted for salted provisions." In his own remarks, Sauer concluded that the outbreak "arose solely from the carelessness of the men, in going with wet feet. The water was a collection of melted snow, very cold. The weather hazy and damp." Roebeck had concluded that the scurvy outbreak was primarily linked to the men drinking "very dirty rainwater that had been collected on deck."[52]

The Billings crew tried all possible treatments, just as the Second Kamchatka Expedition had: "We had malt, hops, and a considerable quantity of essence of spruce; and beer was brewed for the benefit of all hands, especially the sick. Berries were also administered, and every antiscorbutic that we could procure; but we did not perceive any good arose from it." With little result from the traditional remedies, many of which had been used unsuccessfully since the seventeenth century, Sauer suggested an alternate solution: "Thinking the best way to guard against it was to copy the natives in their mode of living, I made the chief part of my diet consist of raw fish, muscles, and limpets; using, instead of tea in the morning, a tea-spoonful of essence of spruce in a small tea-kettle full of boiling water; and in the evening, we boiled beer with berries, sugar, and pepper, which, with the addition of some corn-brandy, was our substitute for punch." By the end of 1790, however, scurvy still overwhelmed his crew despite their preparations. By February 1791, "it raged with unabashed violence; . . . we sometimes buried three men in one day; and the most athletic in appearance were the earliest victims."[53]

The failure to maintain the crew's health was not from lack of interest in local habits. Merck mentioned while on Kamchatka that the Indigenous communities relied on "winter provisions" of "dried, frozen, or salted fish, several kinds of berries, strong leek, and here in addition *sarana* among other kitchen herbs. So long as these provisions last, these people know nothing of scurvy, not even when in spring (a time when many incline toward laziness because of normally easier access to provisions) the rest of the winter provisions are supplemented with bark peeled from larch trees and willows."[54] Sarychev noted the Iukagirs had their own prophylactic: "red bilberries mashed with dried fish, and the fat of fish. . . . It is reputed to be very salutary against the scurvy."[55] Just like the Second Kamchatka Expedition, interest in local cures failed to save the Russia crew from another disaster in the Pacific. Nonetheless, the Billings Expedition contributed to knowledge of scurvy treatments through the sacrifices of its crew.

The Billings Expedition may have begun as a response to the political challenge generated by Cook's third voyage, but the narratives it produced undermined the idea of Russia's success. It generated new navigation charts and maps for the Russian government, but it did not meet its loftier aspirations. The Second Kamchatka Expedition had cooperated with Linnaeus and demonstrated the Russian Empire's value to the progress of science, but the Billings Expedition came up far short and only added new criticism by revealing Russia's limited impact on its far east and North Pacific possessions.

The Billings Expedition relied on an ad hoc response to scurvy, first using known local remedies and then trying any potential solution without great success. The next major expedition, Russia's first circumnavigation (1803–1806), approached scurvy more deliberately with advanced preparations. The doctor accompanying the voyage, Georg Heinrich von Langsdorff, who had trained at the University of Göttingen and was a member of the Russian Academy of Sciences, was a product of a long line of German physicians in Russian service. He would be given responsibility for implementing a prophylactic treatment to prevent scurvy during the circumnavigation, but it was not a therapy of his design. The decision appears to have been made by the voyage's leader, Adam Johann Ritter von Krusenstern. Krusenstern was born in Estonia in 1770, and joined the Russian Navy in 1787. He then joined the British Royal Navy in 1793, staying for six years before returning to Russian service. In the Royal Navy, Krusenstern became acquainted with the so-called Cook method of preventing scurvy outbreaks and also became a student of other well-known explorations of the Pacific, including several French and British explorers: Jean François de Galaup, comte de Lapérouse; Samuel Wallis, Philip Carteret, and Louis Antoine de Bougainville.[56] From this practical knowledge, Krusenstern was careful to implement the best practices available. It was not the medical community, but rather the naval one, that successfully brought the new scurvy prophylactics to Russia.

When Krusenstern's two ships departed St. Petersburg in 1803 on his great expedition, he was fully aware of the importance of food preparation. He wrote that he promised to preserve "the health of the crew, from the use of sourcrout and cranberry juice," as well as tea and sugar, which was well known to be a "healthy and antiscorbutic beverage," reflecting his implementation of the British naval regulations. Unfortunately, "sufficient attention had not been paid to the choice of casks, the consequence of which was, that a good deal of the provision was destroyed," including two-thirds of his sauerkraut. Beyond the food, Krusenstern was careful with the overall health of the crew. He provided "an ample provision" of "clothes and linen, as well for warm as cold weather" and was pleased "to see an inclination to cleanliness in all of them." To guarantee healthful behavior, he "examined them twice a week, took notice of their linen and clothes, and particularly of the cleanliness of their persons." The preparations may have helped the crew avoid a crisis in the Atlantic, allowing them to reach Hawai'i without incident. Upon his arrival there, Krusenstern noted that "my people are healthy; but in a long voyage like this, during which, except the first weeks after our departure from Brazil, they had had no other provisions than salt meat."[57]

Krusenstern's preparations, however, failed to inspire sweeping reforms against scurvy in Russia's Pacific. Visiting Kamchatka and later Russian America, Krusenstern and Langsdorff would be horrified by the pervasiveness of scurvy throughout Russian territory. One of the ships of the Russian American Company he encountered, the *Maria*, was filled with a scurvy-stricken crew living in miserable conditions. Krusenstern found them living in "shocking, disgusting state, . . . nearly all appeared to labour under incurable scorbutic and venereal sores, although they had been ten months on shore, and had enjoyed the assistance of the surgeon of [the outposts at] St. Peter and St. Paul." The causes were clear to Krusenstern—that is, the "extremely pernicious" climate of the north Pacific, coupled with "filthiness and laziness." Although these causes looked back to the most traditional ideas of the cause of scurvy, Krusenstern knew that proper food could be a cure, leading him to inspect the available provisions, which was only salted meat: "On opening a cask so disgusting and pestilential a smell took possession of the hold as compelled me instantly to quit it."[58] The lack of antiscorbutics, either traditional or more recent options (like cranberry juice), coupled with the miasmatic air of rancid meat, left little chance of recovery for the victims.

Krusenstern left Kamchatka for his diplomatic mission in Japan, leaving the other ship, the *Neva*, under the direction of his second-in-command, Iurii Fedorovich Lisianskii. Born in Ukraine, Lisianskii also joined the Russian Navy at a young age and followed this experience with six years in the British Royal Navy. Lisianskii was given the task of inspecting Russian America, from the Aleutian Islands south to California. Throughout the voyage along the coast of Alaska, scurvy was an endemic problem, partially caused by the lack of proper provisions from Kamchatka. The crew took advantage of a short stay on the island of St. Paul to gather "fresh provisions for our diseased and half-starved crew," the flesh of sea-bear and birds' eggs. As Langsdorff noted: "It was indeed not a little striking to see the change that a few days of better feeding made in these miserable people. The scurvy visibly decreased, and a vivacity and joviality hitherto unknown was observable among them." This was unfortunately a temporary solution, however, as the "most afflicted" with the disease would be left behind on Kodiak Island and were replaced with local men. Their provisions were restocked with fresh fish and "good water"[59]

Scurvy became an inescapable part of the crew's life for the rest of their voyage, in a remarkable change from the first half of the voyage from St. Petersburg to Kamchatka. Langsdorff believed that wintering on Sitka Island left the crew with little chance to escape, despite having selected "the youngest and most healthy men" for the voyage (figure 6.2). It was their lifestyle on the island that was to blame, as the crew had "not the remotest idea of cleanliness," and frequently "came home in the evening wet through, perhaps covered with snow, and lay down upon the beds in their wet cloaths, . . . without any one appearing to think of the pernicious consequences that might ensue." As a result, scurvy "shewed itself first by debility, listlessness, and melancholy; inflammatory spots,

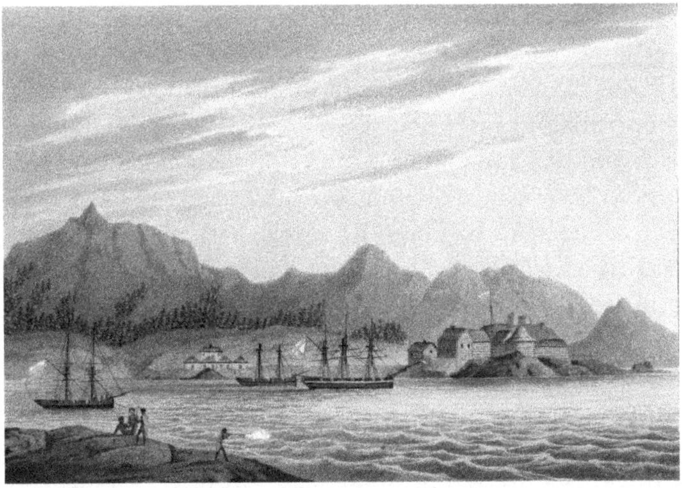

FIGURE 6.2. Krusenstern's circumnavigation highlighted Russia's progress in North America, featuring the new settlement in Sitka. "Harbour of New Archangel in Sitca or Norfolk Sound," Rare Book Division, The New York Public Library, New York Public Library Digital Collections, accessed June 9, 2024, https://digitalcollections.nypl.org/items/510d47d9-7b43-a3d9-e040-e00a18064a99.

sometimes larger, sometimes smaller, then appeared on the legs from the knees to the toes."[60] The argument that melancholy preceded physical symptoms appeared frequently in the eighteenth century, although in this case its inclusion seemed to be as much for narrative effect as a physical description of the symptoms.

At this point, Langsdorff suggested the Russian American Company's resistance toward treatment was the key for the lack of treatment, which did place the blame on the company rather than on the state or himself as the physician on the scene. He tried the traditional solutions, including an attempt to establish a "dry, warm, airy, and clean apartment allotted to the sick," but his voice "was too weak to be heard." Failing that, he tried better food, "representing that sugar, rice, molasses, and other wholesome kinds of nourishment, were of more importance to the sick than medicine, and that a wholesome liquor might be made for them to drink from spruce-fir with molasses." Unfortunately, the company's managers rejected this offer as well, suggesting that it "must be a pretty doctor who would cure his patients with good eating and drinking, instead of medicine." Sadly, it is also unlikely the local medicines would have provided any relief. As Langsdorff noted, the available medicine consisted of "steel-filings, juniper-berries, essence of spruce, of which there were several poods, calcareous powders, and other things of the same kind; not an emetic or purgative medicine, no opium, nor any preparations of mercury, not any in short of the most important and useful medicines."[61]

The circumnavigation differed from the earlier academy expeditions. The Russian Navy led the Second Kamchatka and Billings Expeditions, but medical decisions had been led by the naturalists and physicians, whereas Krusenstern set the course for scurvy mitigation instead of his physician. This may explain why the search for local cures, which had been so prominent in the earlier expeditions, did not appear to interest the crew of the circumnavigation. If the earlier expeditions created opportunities for scientific discoveries, gathering insight on local products and potential commodities, and uncovered regional medical treatments, this nineteenth-century undertaking focused on imperial control over North America and foreign trade in the Pacific Ocean as its main objectives. It was not the only change, but it does suggest that improving health and mastering the climate did not hold the same priority for the state as it had in the eighteenth century.

Guthrie wrote about Russia's climate one final time, in a manuscript that remained unfinished when he died in 1807. In its introduction, Guthrie stated that he undertook this project to respond to Russia's critics who still believed in climate determinism, those who argued that "a People living under rigorous Climate, and despotic government with a state of compleat Vassalage, . . . [led] a life of Langour, Sufferance and Misery, in perfect ignorance and Barbarity." In response to those critics, Guthrie offered "real and actual observations" of those "living under frigid Climate, and absolute government, who resembled the Freeman of Greece, than the desponding laws which had represented him. That he is endowed, with a Sensible gayty, dexterity, that he is born a Musician, passionately fond of a line of Poetry, of Amusements, and Stage plays."[62] Much of his text was devoted to the connection between contemporary Russia and classical Greece, with a particular focus on the arts. For Guthrie, Russia's rich cultural tradition disproved any belief in climate determinism; the cold climate did not have a negative impact on Russians.

Furthermore, Guthrie discussed at length the importance of the bania for Russians of all ranks, once again arguing that the extreme heat prevented the danger of putrefaction in the body. Russia's bania was "a Vapour Bath which a man must be accustomed to from his infancy to relish or you are obliged whilst in it to breath Vapour instead of Air, raised by throwing Water on red hot stones." The benefit for all Russians was clear, as "this practice of hardening men by exactly the same process that we harden steel, has a happy effect on the Russian Constitution, gradually inured to it from the day of their Birth for it is to the Banoi (as they calle it) a Woman repairs, with her in fact the very day she is delivered and often repairs there whilst in Labour to facilitate delivery."[63] His arguments closely resembled those offered on the Second Kamchatka Expedition, if not earlier. Despite his multiple publications on Russians' ability to manage their environment, even at the dawn of the nineteenth century, Guthrie felt it was necessary to reiterate these same ideas.

Guthrie's intention to prove once again that the Russian Empire had overcome its climate challenge was not unnecessary. Critics of Russia's management of its empire continued to emphasize the state's failure both to improve the health of its population and to utilize its resources more effectively. Some of these critics were foreign like Lesseps, but increasingly some worked for the Russian government, like Sauer and Krusenstern. Texts from both the Billings Expedition and the circumnavigations relied on familiar tropes to describe and classify the peoples of the North Pacific and observed common diseases that still included scurvy, syphilis, and smallpox. Even if these expeditions were intended to highlight the empire's successes, the similarity of the images, language, and ideas produced during these voyages with that of the Second Kamchatka Expedition produced an impression that little had changed in decades.

An additional challenge emerged at the dawn of the century for Russia's physicians beyond the empire's critics. Disease theory was changing. At the beginning of the eighteenth century, putrefaction was widely accepted as a major cause of disease, making a cold climate extremely dangerous. As contagious or miasmatic vectors for disease transmission were more widely accepted, the climate was less of a particular risk. The multiple theories of the origin of the Russian catarrh demonstrated the progress of those new ideas by the 1780s. This raised a new question for the new century: If the climate was not the cause of Russia's unhealthy empire, then what was to blame? Critics of the empire may have blamed the tsar and his government for Russia's mismanagement of its land and peoples. Russia's defenders, like Guthrie, not only had to highlight the empire's achievements in public health but also had to respond to these political issues. Guthrie's intention with his final manuscript was to address both, but sadly, it remained unfinished at the time of his death. When Guthrie was writing in the first decade of the new century, however, all the information necessary to offer a defense of Russia's successes existed. It is not hard to understand why no one immediately accepted the task following Guthrie's death. The general confusion of the Napoleonic era, including the French invasion of Russia in 1812, was not an auspicious time to produce a comprehensive history of the empire's climate and its progress in public health. There may have been new interest in the consequences of a cold climate after 1812, but the decimation of the Grand Armée was now far more relevant than Russia's imperial challenges.

Epilogue

Alexander Crichton was born in Scotland in 1763, studied at the University of Edinburgh as an undergraduate, and conducted clinical work in London before receiving his medical doctorate from the University of Leiden in 1785. In 1803, he was hired by Tsar Aleksander I (r. 1801–1825) to serve as his personal physician. The appointment was not a surprise. Crichton's father enjoyed a lengthy business relationship with Dr. John Rogerson, Catherine the Great's personal physician; Rogerson recommended Crichton for the appointment.[1] At Edinburgh, Crichton studied anatomy with Dr. John Bell, who had served on three tsarist embassies earlier in the century. During his clinical work in London, Crichton studied with Dr. William Fordyce, one of the men involved in the export of rhubarb from Russia, which had made him a personal acquaintance of both John Bell and James Mounsey, who was Elizaveta Petrovna's physician.[2] It was not only the social network that had brought Crichton to Aleksander's awareness, as Crichton's professional reputation had been established by his *Inquiry Into the Nature and Origin of Mental Derangement* in 1798, positioning him as a leader in the medical field in Britain before his Russian career.[3]

For Crichton, his appointment as the tsar's physician allowed him a range of opportunities in Russia. Along with an apothecary, Konstantin

Kirchov, Crichton established a new business to refine vegetable oil on Aptekarskii Ostrov in 1807.[4] In 1815, alongside two other members of the Academy of Sciences, Crichton edited a volume on the current state of Russian medicine.[5] The following year, he pursued another opportunity—this time launching an investigation of the treatment of consumption (also known as phthisis or tuberculosis, depending on the physician) in St. Petersburg.

Consumption was a cold disease that had yet to gain attention in Russia, but knowledge of the disease advanced elsewhere in Europe. Physicians still employed a nosological approach to analyze disease presentation and transmission vectors at the end of the century, which kept cold diseases as a significant category for study. In 1793, for example, Dr. Thomas Beddoes published *Observations on the Nature and Cure of Calculus, Sea Scurvy, Consumption, Catarrh, and Fever*.[6] It would be the subject of an extensive review in *Medical Commentaries* the following a year, a publication of which all of the Edinburgh physicians working in Russia remained subscribers, including Matthew Guthrie.[7] Beddoes employed a nosological approach to address the four major cold diseases. All four were the result of too much exposure to cold moist air, although Beddoes argued the varied nature of the symptoms required varied approaches to treatment. He accepted that putrefaction led to the formation of calculus "stones" (of all sorts) and scurvy. For both, his cure was a compound of "vegetable alkali" to break up the putrefaction. He was aware, however, the cost would be prohibitive for the "poor." Thus, he provided them an alternate, "fossil alkali," a compound prepared from crushed natron mixed with soap to make a pill. For either option, if the patient also had a fever, "aromatics, extract of Peruvian bark, &c. may be added."[8]

Both of the pulmonary diseases resulted from an alteration of the level of oxygen in the blood, whether too much (consumption) to too little (catarrh). Consumption could be solved by treating the patient with a diet known to produce scurvy, "salt meat" and an "oily diet," as sailors rarely had consumption despite being in the climate that produced it. In addition, "the supply of oxygen at the lungs must also be diminished, by making the patients breathe air with an additional quantity of azotic or hydrogen airs, and by making them sleep in confined rooms."[9] Catarrh was the result of "sudden alternations of heat and cold; the cold operating, in his opinion, by accumulating irritability, while the inflammation is not produced until the subsequent and too sudden application of heat." The preventative treatment was to wear flannel, "avoid spiritous liquors, warm close rooms, and many bed-clothes."

Even with the ongoing discussions about cold diseases, Crichton's idea to study consumption was a turn from his specialty in mental illness. He lived, however, in Russia during the Napoleonic Era. First, he confronted a personal challenge when the Anglo-Russian War (1807–1812) began after Russia signed the Treaty of Tilsit with France. With his homeland and his employer at war, Crichton opted to remain in Russia and start his new vegetable oil business in St. Petersburg. The timing could be coincidental, but it suggests that his focus was on securing his fortune rather than demonstrating some sort of national loyalty. Britain and Russia returned to friendlier relations in 1812 following the Napoleonic invasion. The subsequent destruction of the Grand Armée inside the Russian Empire demonstrated the need for new studies of the cold and health.

In 1816, Crichton launched a clinical trial for the treatment of consumption in St. Petersburg, following what he later described as a random event. On a walk near his country house outside of the city, he approached a factory that boiled tar as part of the process of producing rope: "I found, to my great surprise, that, although the vapour affected the eyes painfully, yet I breathed the air with perfect ease. In a kind of magazine adjoining to this, where the vapour and odour of boiling tar were weaker, yet strong, the eyes were not affected, and it immediately struck me, that this artificial atmosphere might be of use to a consumptive patient who lived in the neighborhood, and whom I had entirely despaired of curing."[10] Crichton's new therapy was not grounded in medical theory nor was a response to previous treatments. In his summary of these early cases, he offered no evidence that he was a specialist in cold diseases of any kind. Presented with an opportunity to experiment on the public in St. Petersburg from his connection to the tsar, however, Crichton began treating consumptive patients.

Crichton's first case was a thirty-one-year-old man, N., who "of a delicate, lymphatic constitution, and yellowish pale countenance, having the thorax a little flatter than it ought to be, compared with his stature." Following a "common cold" resulting from an apparently ill-timed trip to the bania, N. developed the "symptoms of a tubercular Phthisis" indicated by his "aggravated" cough, the "oppression in his chest," and having "spit a little blood, which soon became very copious." N.'s previous doctors had tried a variety of chemical remedies, most recently "a slight infusion of rose leaves, acidulated with sulphuric acid, with a little opium added," but it had failed to alleviate his symptoms. Crichton sent him to the cable factory. He recounted: "The first day he remained in the tar vapour four hours; and in a very short time after entering the room, he says he experienced a sensation of greater ease on his chest. As the weather was hot, and he had no one there to converse with, he fell asleep, but soon awoke with a headache; still the relief in his breathing was so decided, that he resolved to return to the room on the morrow." Crichton had his patient visit the factory daily and was pleased to observe that "the cough and expectoration had gradually diminished, and at the end of a month he had regained his former strength." N. resumed his normal life in St. Petersburg when his symptoms soon returned, resulting in an agreement with Crichton to begin "fumigating" his room at night with tar.[11]

"Mrs. Fitch, 30 years of age, thin, of a livid complexion, rather flat chested" was Crichton's second tar-cure patient. Crichton believed that a cold she caught during her third pregnancy in the fall of 1815 was the origin of her consumption. This might have been the reason for including her in the trial, as Beddoes had argued pregnant women could not be consumptive.[12] When she consulted him in July 1816, "she appeared . . . in the highest degree consumptive; already a marasmsus had commenced; the cough left her no rest by night or by day; she had a copious exportation of greenish-yellow matter, of a consistence and other apparent qualities of pus." "Believing her case incurable," Crichton ordered tar fumigation for her bedroom, "as her state of extreme debility prevented her from being taken to the cable manufactory." Her recovery surprised Crichton, who allowed her to return to St. Petersburg in September, and she remained in good health a year later.[13]

Encouraged by his two patients' results, Crichton continued his experiment, selecting a women's hospital (St. Petersburg's Hospital for the Poor) and a men's hospital (the Aboukoff, or City Hospital) as his two best options. With permission from Empress Elizaveta Alekseevna, the Hospital for the Poor's trial was supervised by Drs. Bluhm and Roos, who claimed one ward with "four of five beds" for the purpose. Patients in the ward were subjected to "tar fumigation, (pix liquida) . . . three to four times a-day" by placing an "earthen vessel over a lamp or heated iron, to cause a slow volatilization, until the air of the ward be sufficiently impregnated with it." At the City Hospital, Dr. Wochler was assigned, but "the establishment being generally over-crowded with sick, it was not possible to obtain for this purpose more than one small narrow room, where scarcely three beds could be placed."[14] Both hospitals sought patients in the fall of 1816, but only seven patients (six women and one man) had finished their course of treatment by time the trial was ended in June 1817. Of those seven patients, three died but four were declared cured and were subsequently released.

Crichton's work continued. In 1823, he published a lengthier study on the effects of the tar cure on consumptive patients. Since his 1817 pamphlet, new trials proceeded in St. Petersburg and even extended to the Charité Hospital in Berlin under the direction of the Prussian royal physician, Dr. Hufeland. Crichton supervised a third trial in London in 1820 and 1821. The results were mixed. The Berlin trial produced "results nearly as favourable as in the hospital for the poor at St. Petersburgh," with one in twelve cured and those "to be allowed to leave the hospital at their own desire, as one to five." Considering half of his first patients were cured, the 20 percent of the Berlin trial was a significant decline. Even Crichton recognized the London clinic as a failure. For Crichton to continue his experiment, he needed to offer a plausible explanation about the variable results: how patients "in much ruder and colder climates, and which are commonly deemed more injurious to delicate and infirm constitutions" had recovered, whereas those in London's temperate climate had not. No less important was understanding how those "patients in hospitals, and public charities, in cold climates, have advantages which cannot be easily obtained in private practice."[15] Following the destruction of Napoleon's Army, this was a significant issue.

Crichton's 1823 study of the disease was published in London after he left the tsar's service. Crichton had turned his Russian trial into an experiment that would be more relevant for a British audience. The primary issue was not whether the tar cure was effective, but rather why Russia's cold did not produce more illness than Britain's climate? As Crichton noted, "The scrophulous or strumous constitution is more common in northern and middle governments of Russia than in England, and commits greater ravages and disfiguration than are ever witnessed in this country." As the poor treated in St. Petersburg had recovered at a far greater rate than those in Berlin or London, something about the Russian peasants simply worked. At the same time, Crichton was aware that Russia's nobility was facing a similar consumptive crisis as Britain was, "especially those who inhabit the two capitals, and the larger cities, who have adopted the European dress and usages, and are under all the tyranny of European fashion as to late hours and other irregularities, to whom may be added the military in Russia, are becoming every day more and more subject to consumption." He concluded, in agreement with Guthrie and many of his predecessors, that Russian peasant bodies successfully adapted to their climate, producing good health. He remained uncertain, however, which part of their lifestyle was the most important—their warm houses, the bania, or their diet, but one or more of those factors produced people who recovered from cold diseases. Furthermore, once again owing a debt to Guthrie, Crichton argued that Russia's climate was more temperate than expected: "High and frequent winds, one of the richest sources of catarrhal and consequently consumptive cases in this country [Britain], are very rare in the northern parts of Russia."[16]

In the wake of the destruction of Napoleon's army, having Crichton, the tsar's personal physician, suggest Russia's climate was not dangerous may have been difficult to accept in Europe. Indeed, his 1823 text was condemned by the European medical community following its publication.[17] Some of the French medical practitioners who survived the Russian invasion agreed, however. In 1826, for example, Pierre Jean Mauricheau-Beaupré published *A Treatise on the Effects and Properties of Cold*, because "the Russian campaign, the sight of the suffering originating from cold, of which I have been unhappily witness,—I have myself endured,—what I have read, in short, have induced me to reduce to writing various reflections on this agent, which exercises such great influence over man in health and disease, and to add to them a number of facts from my own observation." His conclusions confirmed the work done by the Russian Academy of Sciences nearly a century earlier. In fact, he expressly agreed with Johann Georg Gmelin's work from the Second Kamchatka Expedition: "The Russians are lively, acute, active, industrious and enterprising; they are constantly found cheerful in a temperature which is their element; . . . The rigors of their clime, and their long winters render them eager for amusements; the ordinary pleasures of society, in that season, though less various and brilliant than in happier climes, are not therefore the less keenly relished; their houses resound with them." Mauricheau-Beaupré argued the contentment of Russia's peasants was well known, having been assured by "the French and English, who have lived in Tobolsk and Irkousk, have assured me, that they did not find in those two principal cities of Siberia, that insensibility and apathy so causelessly attributed to the people of cold regions, nor the horrors that seem attached to the very name of that Province. According to Gmelin, the carnival of Tobolsk is very gay, and amid amusement and drunkenness cold is forgotten."[18]

Whereas Jean-Baptiste Chappe-d'Auteroche read Gmelin as a cautionary tale of Russia's inability to manage its empire to care for the health its population, Mauricheau-Beaupré read Gmelin as the Russian medical establishment would have—that is, as the Russians had overcome the dangers of their climate for successful and prosperous lives.

Mauricheau-Beaupré concluded that the extremely high casualty rate for the French army was simply because they were not adapted to the climate: "Not only on account of the untried influence of extreme temperature on individuals born in another climate, but also on account of the fatigues inseparable from traversing long distances, of an irregular, disorderly, and consequently often unhealthful way of life, in short, of a multiplicity of event and circumstances impossible to foresee."[19] The men at work in Russia had been arguing against this conclusion on the climate for decades by the time Mauricheau-Beaupré wrote, but the experience of the French army in Russia's coldness only confirmed that the Russians had long since solved the climatic conditions, but foreigners were still in danger.

A French surgeon, Dominique Jean Larrey, agreed with Mauricheau-Beaupré that Russians may have thrived in the cold but felt unquestionably that the French army was not properly prepared for the climate. He wrote that "it is evidence that cold exercises principally its sedative effects on the brain and nervous system. This is strongly proved by the fact, that, on our return from Moscow, those who were destitute of furred caps or had little hair on their heads, were more obnoxious to cold, the head being deprived of its natural heat." With warm clothing, in other words, the Napoleonic Army's survival rate would have been far greater. This was no small conclusion, as Larrey understood that Montesquieu had observed the "sedative and stupefying influence" of the cold in his *Spirit of Law*; in Larrey's experience in Russia, however, all that it took to overcome the danger of the climate was appropriate dress.[20] Climate was not an unchangeable danger, but rather it was readily manageable (figure E.1).

The failure of the Grand Armeé was a lesson in the importance of studying the climate and its connection to the body. Both Mauricheau-Beaupré and Larrey turned toward earlier work on Russia and its climate to provide a context for the destruction of Napoleon's forces. French critics in the eighteenth century relied on the Russian Academy's expeditions for proof of the climate's danger and the potential threat to exterminate all life in Siberia. French survivors in the early nineteenth century had been persuaded that Russia's peasants might have

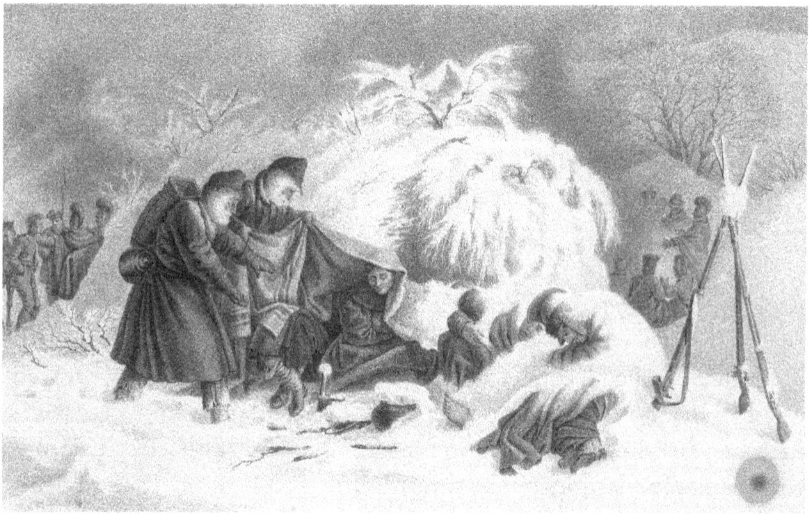

FIGURE E.1. Christian Wilhelm von Faber du Faur, "Frozen to Death," in *Blaetter aus meinem Portfeuille, im Laufe des Feldzugs 1812 in Russland* (Stuttgart: C. F. Autenrieth, 1831–1834). From the British Library Archive.

successfully adapted to the climate and could enjoy good health. It was in fact those men who failed to adopt an appropriate lifestyle, in terms of dress, diet, and activity, who suffered, whether it was elite people living in Russia's cities or the invading Grand Armée. Guthrie believed while he was writing his final text that a defense of Russia's successes was still necessary, but, by the 1820s, recent experiences seemed to have validated the opinion that it was foreigners, not Russian subjects, who suffered from the climate.

The eighteenth-century contributions from the Russian Empire were not solely relevant for the debates on climate. Numerous physicians produced "thick" ethnographic descriptions of the peoples of the empire and those across the North Pacific. Physicians acting as naturalists studied and documented new plants, animals, and minerals. Both groups contributed to the ongoing taxonomic project to classify all these people and materials. Whereas modern scholars focused on the Atlantic or Indian Ocean worlds have analyzed the ways in which European empires transformed the scientific understanding on bodies, this material was being produced not only in tropical environments but also in extremely cold ones. Russia was no less important for European medical knowledge than the Caribbean islands or India were. The less-than-favorable reception of some of the new work produced in the nineteenth century, like Crichton's, should not be counted against its eighteenth-century accomplishments.

If the climate's devastation of the Grand Armée marked an inauspicious start to the nineteenth century, it is only that much more important to remember Russia's genuine achievements in the previous century. The establishment of the Academy of Sciences supported the taxonomic project. The discovery of new materials, plants, and minerals increased Europe's pharmacopeia. The decades of study on scurvy contributed to Europe's ability to improve therapies for disease. Catherine the Great's smallpox inoculation campaign did improve the health of the empire. Russia managed multiple plague outbreaks and adopted quarantine strategies that prevented the spread of the disease to Europe. The lesson may be that the general impression of Russia and its climate owes more to the prevalence of the humorally influenced language that dominated travel narratives than to any of its material accomplishments. Once Russia became fixed as a cold place in the European imagination, no one may have been able to envision it as a healthy state. French critics may have offered dire predictions, but the only group that faced those consequences were the French themselves. The Russians, as they always had, continued to prosper.

Acknowledgments

This book began as an accident. For my first sabbatical from University of Hawai'i, I planned my new project to be a study of tobacco consumption in the Russian Empire. That idea was a result of reading travel narratives about Russia, which provided some insight into imperial habits that I had not expected. I have a vivid memory of working my way through Johann Gottlieb Georgi's multivolume description of the empire and thinking that his extensive comments about the populations should really be its own book. The other part was that what I was teaching at Hawai'i had evolved. One of my courses was on Renaissance and Reformation Europe, which first I taught as a course on gender in the early modern era, then as a course on sexuality, and then as a course on early modern medicine. Driven by student interest, I started teaching history of medicine more often, adding courses on early modern medicine, colonial medicine, and the history of human diseases. After my sabbatical in 2013–2014 (when I was conducting the research on tobacco that eventually turned into *Enterprising Empires*), I realized that the descriptions of the empire I had been reading fit into a discussion with all the colonial medicine texts I was using in class. The Russian Empire's absence in those studies was confusing, because its physicians were produced by the same medical schools and published in the same eighteenth-century journals. Addressing that gap became the motive for this book.

Some of the research for this book was completed during my sabbatical from Hawai'i in 2013–2014. I still owe thanks to the History Department and the College of Arts and Humanities at the University of Hawai'i at Mānoa for providing that opportunity. Hawai'i also provided leave in 2017–2018 so that I could have a full year to work on this book on a fellowship at the Tanner Humanities Center at the University of Utah. It was a productive year, but finishing this book was delayed for some unexpected reasons, beginning with leaving my job at Hawai'i for my current position at Weber State University. A return to the archives in Scotland in 2018 raised some new questions to consider, as I wondered if the physicians' networks and private exchanges were as central to this story as their publications. My intention to return to the archives in the summer of 2020 to answer that question was derailed by the COVID-19 pandemic. When I finally returned to the archives in the United Kingdom in the summer of 2022 and then again in the spring of 2023, I finished the research, but the enforced delay in completing the book allowed its focus to evolve. It is far better because of this extended delay, but I never expected to take this long on a book that I thought was nearly finished in 2018.

I am greatly indebted to all those who helped over the past decade. This includes staffs of the National Archives in Kew, the British Library, the Royal Society for Arts Archive, the Wellcome Library, the Bedfordshire Archive, the National Records of Scotland, and the National Library of Scotland. Equally important may be the opportunities to discuss this project in multiple presentations since 2014 at conferences and several invited lectures. It started at University of Hawaiʻi after my long-ago sabbatical, then at Weber State and Utah State University on two separate trips in 2016, University of Toronto in 2018, and Ohio State University in 2024. I also benefited from the opportunity to present at the Forum on Early-Modern Empires and Global Interactions in 2014; Social History of Medicine's biennial meeting at University of Oxford later that year; Association for Slavic, East European, and Eurasian Studies (ASEEES) in 2015 and via Zoom in 2020; the Association for the History of Medicine's annual meeting in Los Angeles in 2018; and the Study Group on Eighteenth Century Russia in 2022. I thank all the participants of those panels for their suggestions and advice over the years.

The final version of this book also benefited from my participation in a series of different workshops in the past decade. In 2014, Fran Bernstein, Chris Burton, and Dan Healey organized a meeting at Oxford on Continuity and Change in Russian Therapy and graciously invited me to join even though I had only just begun working on the history of medicine. I will always remember the suggestion made at the Russian History Desert Workshop held at Arizona State in 2019, organized by Laurie Manchester, for encouraging me to think about reorganizing the book from its history of disease orientation to instead foreground the multiple narratives generated by the academy's expeditions in the eighteenth century. Andy Bruno and Pey-Yi Chu invited me to join their workshop at the University of Illinois on Climate and Society in Eurasia in 2020 and 2021, which nudged me toward the final version of this book. Johanna Conterio invited me to join her workshop on Ecologies of Health and Disease in Eurasia held at the Oslo School of Environmental Humanities, which provided an opportunity to rethink the role of Linnaeus and his taxonomy.

No less important were the opportunities created by organizing workshops and panels that allowed me to think through this material in different contexts. Trish Starks and I held a series of panels at ASEEES on the history of senses that became a volume, including my first article on the experience of the cold in Russia. In 2018, I worked alongside Jane Hacking and Jeff Hardy to organize Asia in the Russian Imagination at University of Utah, where I presented an early version of chapter 1. In 2023, Alison Smith, Trish Starks, and I held a workshop on the cold in Russia at University of Toronto, which provided an opportunity for me to receive feedback on a draft of the introduction of this book. I also have to thank the other fellows at the Tanner Humanities Center in 2017–2018, as enjoying the time to develop and discuss the ideas of the first version of this book was particularly essential to the final product. Kevin Coe from Communications, Jeremy Rosen and Jessica Straley from English, and Danielle Olden from History all contributed toward a productive year.

There are too many people to thank who have influenced my thoughts and arguments in both small and large ways; the audiences for the talks and papers mentioned here is only a partial acknowledgment. Trish Starks and Alison Smith have read and commented on the entire manuscript more than once. Clare Griffin read the first two chapters several years ago, providing some incisive comments that led to one of the major shifts in the book's focus. My colleagues at Weber State have graciously let me ramble on about climate and disease over the past six years and helped push this book over the finish line. I am appreciative that James Almeida and Stephen Francis willingly read a new draft of the introduction at the eleventh hour. I am grateful for all their support.

My first thoughts on humoral bodies in the Russian Empire were published in an article, "Humoral Bodies in Cold Climates," included in *Russian History through the Senses: From 1700 to the Present*, edited by Matthew P. Romaniello and Tricia Starks, for Bloomsbury Academic in 2016. The first part of chapter 6 shares material with my article, "The Influential Influenza: The 'Russian Catarrh' Pandemic of 1781–1782," which was published in the *Journal of the History of Medicine and Allied*

Sciences 79 (2024). I should also thank the New York Public Library for its extraordinary digital collections, which greatly enhanced the final version of this text.

Finally, this book has traveled a lengthy road toward publication. I owe a great debt to Amy Farranto, Christine Worobec, and the reader for the press for their guidance. The final version of the monograph is much stronger for their recommendations.

None of this would have been possible without the support of my family on the East Coast and in Utah. My greatest debt of appreciation is always for Paul Hibbeln, because his support and encouragement make everything possible.

Notes

Introduction

1. Crichton, *Practical Observations*, 50, 21.

2. Sydenham, *Whole Works*, 5, 6.

3. The work on cold diseases at the end of the century included Mudge, *Radical and Expeditious Cure*; and Beddoes, *Observations on the Nature and Cure*.

4. Among the instances when this argument appeared, see "Rondeau to Harrington," 30 December 1738, TNA, SP 91/22, fols. 317–18; and "Cathcart to Suffolk," 30 December 1771/10 January 1772, TNA, SP 91/89, fols. 21–27.

5. For a general history of scurvy, see Carpenter, *History of Scurvy*. For Russia specifically, Bartlett, "Britain, Russia, and Scurvy."

6. Kupperman, "Fear of Hot Climates"; Kupperman, "Puzzle of the American Climate"; Harrison, *Climates and Constitutions*.

7. Rutman and Rutman, "Of Agues and Fevers"; Cates, "The 'Seasoning'"; Merrens and Terry, "Dying in Paradise."

8. Morgan, *Laboring Women*; Manen, "Preventative Medicine in the Dutch Slave Trade."

9. On the Little Ice Age, see Appleby, "Epidemics and Famines"; Fagan, *Little Ice Age*; Parker, *Global Crisis*; Sundberg, *Natural Disaster*.

10. Pokrovskii, *Tomsk 1648–1649 gg.*; Kivelson, "Devil Stole His Mind."

11. Brikner, "Chuma v Moskve."

12. Charters, "Disease, Wilderness, Warfare"; Zilberstein, *Temperate Empire*; Zeheter, *Epidemics, Empire, and Environments*; Piper, *When Disease Came to This Country*.

13. For an introduction, see Bishop, "English Physicians in Russia."

14. Boyle, *New Experiments and Observations*.

15. Lind, *Treatise of the Scurvy*.

16. Romaniello, *Enterprising Empires*.

17. I have been influenced by Schiebinger, *Plants and Empire*; Cook, *Matters of Exchange*, esp. chap. 7; Gänger, "World Trade in Medicinal Plants." On the process in Europe, see Cooper, *Inventing the Indigenous*.

18. Daston and Lunbeck, *Histories of Scientific Observation*; Pender and Struever, *Rhetoric and Medicine*.

19. Chakrabarty, *Provincializing Europe*; Pratt, *Imperial Eyes*; Dainotto, *Europe (In Theory)*.

20. Bleys, *Geography of Perversion*; Cheek, *Sexual Antipodes*.

21. Raj, *Relocating Modern Science*; Wisecup, *Medical Encounters*; Gómez, *Experiential Caribbean*; Schiebinger, *Secret Cures of Slaves*; Kelton, *Cherokee Medicine, Colonial Germs*; Cagle, *Assembling the Tropics*; Barca, *Yellow Demon of Fever*; Küçük, *Science Without Leisure*; Kananoja, *Healing Knowledge in Atlantic Africa*.

22. Chaplin, *Subject Matter*; Kidd, *Forging of Races*; Earle, *Body of the Conquistador*; Curran, *Anatomy of Blackness*; Hogarth, *Medicalizing Blackness*; Block, *Colonial Complexions*; Seth, *Difference and Disease*.

23. Smith, "'Freedom to Choose a Way of Life'"; and Smith, "Movement and the Transformation."

24. On the European commentary, see Wolff, *Inventing Eastern Europe*; and Poe, *A People Born to Slavery*.

25. Jones, *Empire of Extinction*; Vermeulen, *Before Boas*.

26. Historians of medicine who work on the modern era are often uncomfortable with the application of the term "public health" before the late nineteenth century, where it gained a particular meaning and framework. When historians of the early modern era discuss state actions to improve the general health and well-being of the population, however, they describe this as public health. See Blum, *Strength in Numbers*; Cody, *Birthing the Nation*; Bowers, *Plague and Public Health*; Chase-Levenson, *Yellow Flag*.

27. Alexander, *Bubonic Plague in Early Modern Russia*; Kuxhausen, *From the Womb to the Body Politic*; Robarts, *Migration and Disease*.

28. Griffin, *Mixing Medicines*.

29. The exceptions are Romaniello, "Humoral Bodies in Cold Climates"; Herzberg et al., *Russian Cold*.

30. Bentham, *Fragment on Government*, 93.

31. Guthrie, "Dissertation."

32. Tansey, "Life and Works," 251, 253.

1. Experiencing Climate, Observing People

1. Fletcher, *Of the Russe Common Wealth*, fols. B3–B3v.

2. Fagan, *Little Ice Age*; Parker, *Global Crisis*; Sundberg, *Natural Disaster*.

3. "William Prideaux to John Thurloe," 16 September 1654, in Birch, *Collection of the State Papers*, vol. 2, 607.

4. "Prideaux to Thurloe," 16 December 1654, in Birch, *Collection of the State Papers*, vol. 3, 26–27.

5. For an example, see Harrison, *Medicine in an Age of Commerce and Empire*; Chase-Levenson, *Yellow Flag*.

6. "Prideaux to Thurloe," 16 September 1654, in Birch, *Collection of the State Papers*, vol. 2, 607–8.

7. Earle, *Body of the Conquistador*, 26–30; see also Harrison, *Climates and Constitution*, 25–57.

8. On the importance of climate, see Miller, "'Airs, Waters, and Places'"; on the persistence of the nonnaturals in eighteenth-century medicine, see Riley, "The Medicine of the Environment"; and Emch-Dériaz, "The Non-Naturals Made Easy."

9. This method of description facilitated diagnosing patients and providing care through correspondence rather than needing in-person examinations.

Among the works on this topic, see Louis-Courvoisier and Mauron, "'He found me very well."

10. Ehninger, "On Systems of Rhetoric."

11. The intersection of popular and medical knowledge is a well-trod subject; see for example, Cole, "In Search of a New Mentality."

12. "Republic of Letters" is a long-established concept to describe correspondence networks among educated elites in early-modern Europe; see Daston, "Ideal and Reality."

13. On Boyle's connection to Samuel Collins, see Loewenson, "Works of Robert Boyle"; and Hunter and Davis, "The Making of Robert Boyle's 'Free Enquiry.'"

14. Boyle, *New Experiments*, 521, 529, 532.

15. Bay, *Beriberi in Modern Japan*.

16. Lomax, "Difficulties in Diagnosing Infantile Scurvy"; on Russian doctors early understanding of scurvy, see Petrov, "Tsinga i bor'ba."

17. For a discussion of Glisson and his assistants, see Birken, "Dissenting Tradition in English Medicine"; for the broader context, see Newton, "Diagnosing Rickets in Early Modern England."

18. Tikhomirov, *Pravila o sposobe vrachevaniia*. The "English disease" remained rickets common name in Russia throughout the nineteenth century; see Zhukovskii, *Rakhit*; Gal'perin and Tarkhanov, *Angliiskaia boliezn' rakhit*.

19. Donkin, *Manna*, 98–103.

20. [Dr. Skinner], *Some Observations*, 4–5.

21. Dale's text was a supplement to his 1693 pharmacopoeia. Dale, *Pharmacologiae*, 252–53.

22. "Letter from D. Wolfe about Polish manna," 1760, RSA, PR/GE/110/9/15.

23. Collins, *Present State*, 13, 23, 13.

24. Collins, *Present State*, 35–37, 106, 67–68, 96–97.

25. Collins, *Present State*, 42–43.

26. Collins, *Present State*, 76–77.

27. Collins, *Present State*, 78.

28. Boterbloem, *Fiction and Reality of Jan Struys*, 53–103.

29. Struys, *Perilous and most Unhappy Voyages*, 117, 136, 137.

30. Struys, *Perilous and most Unhappy Voyages*, 139–40.

31. Struys, *Perilous and most Unhappy Voyages*, 136, 135, 140.

32. Avril, *Travels Into divers Parts*, 135.

33. Avril, *Travels Into divers Parts*, 116–17, 120, 126.

34. Avril, *Travels Into divers Parts*, 86.

35. Earle, *Body of the Conquistador*, 141–42.

36. Avril, *Travels Into divers Parts*, 163–64.

37. Avril, *Travels Into divers Parts*, 164.

38. Avril, *Travels Into divers Parts*, 85, 116.

39. On the operation of the Royal Society, see Porter, "Early Royal Society."

40. Crull, *Account of the Antient*, 2, 146–47.

41. Crull, *Account of the Antient*, 139–40, 145.

42. Crull, *Account of the Antient*, 152; see also 132–33.

43. Crull, *Account of the Antient*, 15.

44. Crull, *Account of the Antient*, 41–42.
45. Crull, *Account of the Antient*, 79.
46. Crull, *Account of the Antient*, 80–81, 81.
47. Allison, *Account of a Voyage*.
48. "Journal of a voyage to Archangel and back under Capt. W. Baker, 1702," BL, Sloane MS 3237, fols. 39–47b.
49. Romaniello, *Enterprising Empires*, 29–37.
50. Ssu-ming, "E-lo-ssu kuan"; Monahan, *Merchants of Siberia*, 55, 181–82.
51. Dmytryshyn, "Iurii Krizhanich"; and Slezkine, "Sovereign's Foreigners."
52. Both men wrote narratives that were translated into English. Brand, *Journal of the Embassy*; Ides, *Three Years Travels*.
53. Ides, *Three Years Travels*, 75.
54. "Ostiak" was a broad label for several groups of distinct Siberian peoples, including Khanty, Selkup, or Ostiak-Samoyeds. Brand, *Journal of the Embassy*, 39.
55. Ides, *Three Years Travels*, 20.
56. Brand, *Journal of the Embassy*, 47. "Tungus" is another broad label for several groups of Siberian peoples, including Manchus, Evenks, and Evens.
57. Brand, *Journal of the Embassy*, 48.
58. Purdue, "Boundaries, Maps, and Movement."
59. Brand, *Journal of the Embassy*, 48–49, 51.
60. Brand, *Journal of the Embassy*, 40–41.
61. European travelers' expectations for sexual access to Indigenous populations was not specific to Russia. Bleys, *Geography of Perversion*, 63–109; Cheek, *Sexual Antipodes*, esp. chaps. 4–6.

2. Training Physicians, Exchanging Information

1. Among the works on this topic, see Debus, "Chemists, Physicians, and Changing Perspectives"; Cook, "History of Medicine."
2. Chaplin, *Subject Matter*, 81. This discussion also reflects the idea of the conception of the body reflecting cultural constructions; see Butler, "Foucault and the Paradox of Bodily Inscriptions."
3. On Russia's reliance on apothecaries and chemical experiments, see Griffin, *Mixing Medicines*.
4. Lindeboom, *Herman Boerhaave*, 4.
5. Emch-Dériaz, "Non-Naturals Made Easy," 134–59.
6. Cook, *Matters of Exchange*, 149–51.
7. Cook, *Matters of Exchange*.
8. For a further discussion, see Rosner, *Medical Education in the Age of Improvement*, 2; Cunningham, "Medicine to Calm the Mind," 49.
9. Sydenham, *Whole Works*. On nosology as a practice, see DeLacy, "Nosology, Mortality, and Disease Theory."
10. Lindeboom, *Herman Boerhaave*, 8–9.
11. DeLacy, *Germ of an Idea*, 3.
12. Goslings, "Leiden and Edinburgh," 10.
13. DeLacy discusses this turn in medical practice more broadly; see DeLacy, *Germ of an Idea*, 171.

14. Knoppers, "Visits of Peter the Great," 66-67.

15. Cunningham, "Medicine to Calm the Mind," 40-67. On the connection of the British to Göttingen, see Biskup, "University of Göttingen."

16. Broman, *Transformation of German Academic Medicine*, 45.

17. Cunningham, "Medicine to Calm the Mind," 57; Risse, "Clinical Instruction in Hospitals."

18. Broman, *Transformation of German Academic Medicine*, 28–9.

19. Johnson, *Guide for Gentlemen*, 14; see also the discussion in Rosner, *Medical Education*, 38.

20. Bonner, *Becoming a Physician*, 41.

21. Gelfand, *Professionalizing Modern Medicine*, 132.

22. Rosner, *Medical Education*, 52. On Linnaeus's development of his taxonomy, see Larson, *Reason and Experience*, 6–49; and Lindroth, "The Two Faces of Linnaeus."

23. Koerner, *Linnaeus*, 153; see also Stearn, "The Influence of Leyden."

24. Headrick, *When Information Came of Age*, 29. On the tensions between the two men, see also Koerner, *Linnaeus*, 28–29; and Schiebinger, *Nature's Body*, 28, 46–47.

25. For the reception of Buffon's taxonomy in Germany, for example, see Sloan, "Buffon, German Biology."

26. For a discussion of Linnaeus's taxonomy, see Cain, "Logic and Memory"; and Frängsmyr, *Linnaeus*.

27. Rowell, "Linnaeus and Botanists."

28. This argument support Clare Griffin's evidence that Western practitioners willingly adopted local healing practices in Russia; see Griffin, "Russia and the Medical Drug Trade." See also Griffin, *Mixing Medicines*; and Romaniello, "Commodities with Context."

29. Savel'eva, *Katalog knig*. On the reorganization of its library, see also Boterbloem, *Moderniser of Russia*, 102–13.

30. For the history of the Grand Embassy, see Guzevich and Guzevich, *Velikoe posol'stvo*. Peter the Great was no less interested in medicine while in England, where he met the physician and chemist Moses Stringer. Loewensen, "People Peter Met in England," 460–62.

31. Anemone, "Monsters of Peter the Great"; Gordin, "Importation of Being Earnest"; Mazierski, "Cabinet of Frederick Ruysch"; and Vermeulen, *Before Boas*, 47–63.

32. Natochin, "Stanovlenie fiziologii."

33. Alexander, "Medical Developments," 200-201; Driessen van het Reve, "Peter the Great," 150–53.

34. Driessen van het Reve, "Peter the Great," 153; Driessen van het Reve, "Hoe Nicolaas Bidloo (1673/4–1735)."

35. On Bidloo's plans for the hospital and his work in it, see Mirskii, "Moscow Hospital School"; Evangulova, "Rukopisi N. Bidloo"; Kirillov, "Moskva iauzskaia"; and Simonov, "Iatronauchnyi etap."

36. Grmek, "History of Medical Education," 305; Alexander, "Medical Developments," 207–9.

37. By the nineteenth century, it would be more common to spell Areskine's last name as Erskine, but he and his family were Areskine in the seventeenth

and eighteenth centuries. See "Letters and Documents relating to Robert Erskine," NLS, MS 5163. For a brief biography, see Paul, "Scotsmen in Russian Service."

38. For example, Burgess, "Thomas Garvine."

39. For example, "Robert Areskine to Earl of Marr," 29 October 1744, NLS, MS 5163, fols. 27–28; "David Aytoun to Alexander Aytoun," 24 August 1713, NRS, GD1/42/1/23/1; and "George Mackenzie to Dr. Areskine," 10 September 1714, NRS, GD24/1/449. The British government questioned Areskine's connection to the Jacobite rebellions and the influence this might have in Russia, see Dixon, *Britain and Russia*, letters 201, 202, and 205. For the broader history of the Jacobite diaspora, see Murdoch, *Network North*.

40. His family did protest his bequests but did not alter their disposition. "Henry Stirling to Charles Areskine," 7 February 1720, NLS, MS 5163, fols. 57–60; and "Charles Goodfellow to Charles Areskine," 17 February 1719, NLS, MS 5163, fol. 57.

41. Grmek, "History of Medical Education," 306.

42. For example, Leiden had 120 Russian-born students in the eighteenth century, but this number includes students in all disciplines. Hans, "Russian Students at Leyden."

43. Bogdanov, *Materialy dlia biograficheskogo spravochnika russkikh vrachei*. Bogdanov's index was originally published in the 1890s. The other indexes include Chistovich, *Istoriia pervykh meditsynskikh shkol*, and Brückner, *Die Aerzte in Russland*. John T. Alexander relied on Brückner in his *Bubonic Plague*, 37–40, which has a higher number of practitioners than Bogdanov's account.

44. Bonner, *Becoming a Physician*, 21.

45. Rosner, *Medical Education*, 62.

46. Broman, *Transformation of German Academic Medicine*, 28.

47. See for example, Dorwart, "Royal College of Medicine."

48. Dorwart, "Royal College of Medicine"; Geyer-Kordesch, "German Medical Education"; Klein, "Laboratory Challenge."

49. For the rare example of French influence on the academy, see Kuentzel-Witt, "Peter the Great's Intermezzo."

50. On the connection between trade and diplomacy, see Romaniello, *Enterprising Empires*.

51. Hans, "Russian Students," 532–33. The following theses were all written in Latin; I have translated the titles into English for ease of reading.

52. The academy began as the Slavo-Greco-Latin Academy in 1685, founded by two Greek monks who adopted a Jesuit-scientific curriculum. See Chrissidis, *Academy at the Court of the Tsar*.

53. Broman, *Transformation of German Academic Medicine*, 26.

54. Radvoskii, "U istokov anglo-russkikh nauchnykh sviazei"; Thomas, "Sir Hans Sloane"; Bryce, "Russian Collections."

55. Belbourgo, *Collecting the World*.

56. For example, "Linnaeus to Sloane," rec'd 20 December 1737, BL, Sloane MS 4054, fol. 190; and "Boerhaave to Sloane," 17 July 1736, BL, Sloane MS 4054, fol. 248.

57. "Amman to Sloane," 2 March 1736, BL, Sloane MS 4054, fols. 188–89.

58. Catesby in "Amman to Sloane," August 1736, BL, Sloane MS 4054, fols. 297; Moyle and Petty in "Amman to Sloane," 3 June 1738, BL, Sloane MS 4055, fols. 339–40; "Amman to Sloane," 22 July 1739, BL, Sloane MS 4056, fol. 109.

59. This includes "Vigor to Sloane," 21 July 1739, BL, Sloane MS 4056.

60. For context for this discussion, see Erikson, "Linnaeus the Botanist," 63–77; and Schiebinger, *Nature's Body*, 11–39.

61. "Amman to Sloane," August 1736, BL, Sloan MS 4054, fols. 298–99.

62. See the discussion in Larson, *Reason and Experience,* 6–49.

63. For a discussion of the text, see Koroloff, " 'In Imperio Rutheno.' "

64. "Amman to Sloane," 22 April 1738, BL, Sloane MS 4055, fol. 315–16. The text was published the following year, *Stirpium Rariorum in Imperio Rutheno*.

65. "Amman to Sloane," 2 March 1736, BL, Sloane MS 4054, fols. 188–89; "Amman to Sloane," 6 September 1736, Sloane MS 4054, fols. 298–99.

66. "Amman to Linnaeus," 15 September 1736, in Smith, *Selection of the Correspondence*, 2:191–92.

67. "Amman to Linnaeus," 15 November 1737, in Smith, *Selection of the Correspondence*, 2:192–96.

68. On the Iran journey, see Stevens, "John Bell of Antermony."

69. The British consul recommended Bell to the foreign office as a specialist on Eurasian trade in "Claudius Rondeau to Lord Harrington," 17 August 1731, TNA, SP 91/12, fols. 127–28. In 1739, Bell temporarily assumed the role of consul in St. Petersburg following the death of the envoy, Claudius Rondeau, "John Bell to Lord Harrington," 6 October 1739, TNA, SP 91/23, fol. 309.

70. Bell, *Travels from St. Petersburg*.

71. For example, "Letter from John Bell of Antermony," 1 June 1765, NRS, GD253/144/5/1.

72. For Messerschmidt's fieldwork, see Vermeulen, *Before Boas*, 113–24.

73. Bryce, "Russian Collections."

74. Griffin, *Mixing Medicines*, 141–46.

75. *PSZ*, vol. 6, no. 3778, April 1721, 383–87. On the translation project, see Griffin, "In Search of an Audience."

76. *PSZ*, vol. 6, no. 3811, 14 August 1721, 412–13.

77. In 1722, the medical reforms expanded as part of the regulations introduced for the Admiralty that outlined the principles of military medical practice. Haigh, "Design for a Medical Service."

78. Koroloff, " 'In Imperio Rutheno,' " 240–45.

79. Hoffmann, "Strahlenberg," 464.

80. On the history of the two men, see Titova, "Puteshestvie po ukazu Petra I." For Strahlenberg's work, see Strahlenberg, *Das Nord-under Ostliche Theil*, and translated into English as *Historico-Geographical Description*.

81. Some of Messerschmidt's field notes have been published for their ethnographic value, including Napol'skikh, *Udmurtskie materialy*.

82. Sloane, "Account of the elephants teeth," 461, 468.

83. Breyne, "A letter from John Phil. Breyne."

84. Lux and Cook, "Closed Circles or Open Networks?"; Easterby-Smith, "Reputation in a Box"; van den Heuvel et al., "Circles of Confidence."

85. "Amman to Sloane," 20 January 1739, BL, Sloane MS 4056, fols. 28–29.

86. Muller, "Manners and Customs," 70.
87. For an overview of his work, see Vermeulen, *Before Boas*, 108–12.
88. Strahlenberg, *Historico-Geographical Description*, 180, 182.
89. Strahlenberg, *Historico-Geographical Description*, 184.
90. Most would argue that the reception of the physiocrats' understanding of the economy was a later phenomenon, but the underlying principles were already at work. See Konczacki, "Economic and Social Thought"; Alimento, "Entre 'les moeurs des Crétois et les loix de Minos'."
91. Strahlenberg, *Historico-Geographical Description*, 334.
92. Strahlenberg, *Historico-Geographical Description*, 380–81, 382.
93. Strahlenberg, *Historico-Geographical Description*, 402–6.
94. Bernard, *Relation of Grand Tartary*, WL, MS 1143.
95. Bernard, *Recueil du voyages au Nord*.
96. Bernard, *Relation of Grand Tartary*, WL, MS 1143, 6, 7, 8.
97. Bernard, *Relation of Grand Tartary*, WL, MS 1143, 35, 35–36.
98. "Johann Amman to Sloane," 20 January 1739, BL, Sloane MS 4056, fols. 28–29.
99. "Amman to Sloane," 2 March 1736, BL, Sloane MS 4054, fols. 188–89.
100. "Amman to Sloane," 24 January 1741, BL, Sloane MS 4056, fols. 355–56.
101. O'Neill, *Opened Letter*, 4–6.
102. Porter, "Was There a Medical Enlightenment."
103. DeLacy, *Germ of an Idea*, 127.
104. Broman, *Transformation of German Academic Medicine*, 85.
105. On the medical discussion in the *Philosophical Transactions of the Royal Society of London*, see Porter, "Early Royal Society"; and Rusnock, "Correspondence Networks."

3. Describing Kamchatka, Documenting Scurvy

1. For the expedition's contribution to environmental studies, see Jones, *Empire of Extinction*, 21–59. For the expedition's contribution to ethnography, see Vermeulen, *Before Boas*, 131–218. In addition, see also Gibson, *Feeding the Russian Fur Trade*, 13–24; and Black, "G-.F. Müller and the Russian Academy."
2. Koerner, *Linnaeus*, 82–94; Hodacs, "Linnaeans Outdoors," 183–209; Skott, "Human Taxonomies."
3. There was additional pressure to compete with ongoing British efforts in the North Pacific; see Grinëv, "Anglo-Russian Rivalry."
4. *PSZ*, vol. 8, no. 6023, April 17, 1732, 749. The Senate followed this initial *ukaz* with further guidance for the mission on Kamchatka, *PSZ*, vol. 8, no. 6193, September 26, 1732, 932–33.
5. *PSZ*, vol. 8, no. 6041, May 2, 1732, 770–74. See also the instructions from the Senate on the same day: *PSZ*, vol. 8, no. 6042, May 2, 1732, 774–75.
6. *PSZ*, vol. 8, no. 6291, December 28, 1732, 1002–13; Louis Delisle de la Croyère's instructions are article 16, 1012–13.
7. *PSZ*, vol. 9, no. 6351, March 16, 1733, 63–69.
8. *PSZ*, vol. 9, no. 6376, April 21, 1733, 91–92. Other Senate instructions on trade regulations followed involving Okhotsk and Kamchatka, including *PSZ*,

vol. 9, no. 6460, July 26, 1733, 190. On the Treaty of Kiakhta, see Foust, *Muscovite and Mandarin*, 24–67.

9. On the exploration of the northern passage, see Küntzel-Witt, "Eisfrei über den Nordpol?"

10. For the early years of the expedition, see Okhotina-Lind and Meller, *Vtoraia kamchatskaia ekspeditsiia.*

11. Vermeulen focuses on Müller's fieldwork and contribution to ethnography; see Vermeulen, *Before Boas*, 171–94.

12. On Krasheninnikov's contributions, see Shishilov, "K istorii izucheniia materialov S. P. Krasheninnikov."

13. On the scholarly production of the expedition, see Wortman, "Texts of Exploration," 253–56.

14. Rowell, "Linnaeus and Botanists," 17–18.

15. Broman, *Transformation of German Academic Medicine*, 40.

16. Frost, "Vitus Bering and Georg Steller," 3–16; Frost, "Georg Steller and Stepan Krasheninnikov;" Vermeulen, *Before Boas*, 194–96.

17. Steller, *Journal of a Voyage with Bering*, 50.

18. Kuentzel-Witt, "Peter the Great's Intermezzo."

19. For example, de L'Isle, "Extract of a Letter"; and de L'Isle, "Proposal for the measurement."

20. Steller, *Journal of a Voyage with Bering*, 85–86.

21. Gouzévitch, "Delisle Brothers in Russia." The tensions with French *philosophes* will be further discussed in chapter 4.

22. Gibson, *Feeding the Russian Fur Trade*, 72–104; Monahan, *Merchants of Siberia*, 117–23, 202–6; Smith, "Movement and the Transformation," 47–49.

23. Waxell, *American Expedition*, 56.

24. Gibson, *Feeding the Russian Fur Trade*, 46–56.

25. Waxell, *American Expedition*, 70–71, 71.

26. The disastrous ocean voyages of the expedition were detailed in Waxell, *American Expedition*. For an overall assessment, see Grinëv, "Reflections on the Fate"; and Grinëv, "Russian Maritime Catastrophes."

27. "Amman to Sloane," 2 March 1736, BL, Sloane MS 4054, fols. 188–89.

28. "Amman to Sloane," 22 April 1738, BL, Sloane MS 4055, fols. 315–16.

29. "Amman to Sloane," 7 November 1739, BL, Sloane MS 4056, fol. 132.

30. For example, "Gmelin to Linnaeus," 4 February 1746, LCR.

31. For example, "Linnaeus to Gmelin," 15 April 1744, LCR; "Linnaeus to Gmelin," 2 August 1744, LCR; "Gmelin to Linnaeus," 3 September 1744, LCR; "Gmelin to Linnaeus," 20 August 1745, LCR; "Gmelin to Linnaeus," 18 February 1746, LCR; and "Gmelin to Linnaeus," 30 December 1746, LCR. Sexing plants remained a controversial topic across Europe; see, for example, Alston, "Dissertation on the Sexes of Plants," 205–83.

32. For example, "Gmelin to Linnaeus," 3 September 1744, LCR; "Gmelin to Linnaeus," 30 December 1746, LCR; see also Rowell, "Linnaeus and Botanists."

33. Euler, "Extract of a Letter."

34. These include Black, *Russians in Alaska*; Grinëv, *Tlingit Indians in Russian America*; Miller, *Kodiak Kreol*; Vinkovetsky, *Russian America*; and Jones, *Empire of Extinction.*

35. See the discussion in Znamenski, "History with an Attitude."

36. On Linnaeus and Gmelin, see Rowell, "Linnaeus and Botantists." For contemporary reactions to *Flora Sibirica*, see Fothergill, "Account of the Some Observations and Experiments"; and Watson, "Account of the Treatise."

37. Gmelin, *Reise durch Sibirien*; Gmelin, *Voyage en Sibérie*.

38. For example, Gmelin's discussion of Ides's observations, *Voyage en Sibérie*, 2:156–57.

39. "Gmelin to Linnaeus," 4 September 1744, LCR.

40. Gmelin, *Voyage en Sibérie*, 1:232.

41. Gmelin, *Voyage en Sibérie*, 2:183.

42. Skott, "Human Taxonomies," 218–19. Translation by Skott. See also Broberg, "*Homo Sapiens*, Linnaeus's Classification of Man," 165–70, 193–4.

43. Mattson, "Nation-State Science," 321.

44. This includes Sloan, "Buffon, German Biology"; Hudson, "From 'Nation' to 'Race'"; Shoemaker, "How Indians Got to be Red"; Gascoigne, "Royal Society"; Kowner, *From White to Yellow*, esp. chaps. 9–10.

45. Skott, "Human Taxonomies," 219. The tenth edition also gendered the taxonomic system. See Schiebinger, "Why Mammals Are Called Mammals."

46. Koerner, *Linnaeus*, 87. Related to this was their debate over classifying apes; see "Gmelin to Linnaeus," 3 December 1745, LCR.

47. See Geertz, *Interpretation of Cultures*.

48. Gmelin, *Voyage en Sibérie*, 1:327–28.

49. Gmelin, *Voyage en Sibérie*, 1:329.

50. Bleys, *Geography of Perversion*, 63–109; Cheek, *Sexual Antipodes*, esp. chaps. 4–6.

51. Gmelin, *Voyage en Sibérie*, 1:32.

52. Gmelin, *Voyage en Sibérie*, 2:97, 2:98.

53. Gmelin, *Voyage en Sibérie*, 1:129, 1:136.

54. Gmelin, *Voyage en Sibérie*, 2:193, 2:193–94.

55. Cheek, *Sexual Antipodes*, 128–31; Reis, "Impossible Hermaphrodites."

56. Steller, *Steller's History of Kamchatka*, 189, 225.

57. Steller, *Steller's History of Kamchatka*, 191.

58. Steller, *Steller's History of Kamchatka*, 218, 227.

59. Steller, *Steller's History of Kamchatka*, 161, 188.

60. Steller, *Steller's History of Kamchatka*, 218, 219, footnote.

61. Steller, *Steller's History of Kamchatka*, 227–28.

62. Steller, *Steller's History of Kamchatka*, 263, 274.

63. Steller, *Steller's History of Kamchatka*, 218, footnote.

64. This anxiety was common across Europe in the eighteenth century; see Blum, *Strength in Numbers*; Cody, *Birthing the Nation*.

65. "Rondeau to Harrington," 25 June 1737, TNA, SP 91/21, fols. 123–25.

66. "Rondeau to Harrington," 9 September 1738, TNA, SP 91/22, fols. 205–7.

67. "Rondeau to Harrington," 28 October 1738, TNA, SP 91/22, fols. 264–65.

68. "Rondeau to Harrington," 11 November 1738, TNA, SP 91/22, fols. 278–83.

69. "Rondeau to Harrington," 30 December 1738, TNA, SP 91/22, fols. 317–18.

70. For the broader context of Russian views of the Ottomans in this period, see Taki, "Orientalism on the Margins."

71. Sydenham, *Whole Works*, 4–10.

72. "Rondeau to Harrington," 29 September 1739, TNA, SP 91/23, fols. 295-96..

73. "John Bell to Harrington," 6 October 1739, TNA, SP 91/23, fol. 309.

74. "Philip Lernoult to Harrington," 6 October 1739, TNA, SP 91/23, f. 313.

75. "Carmichael to Newcastle," 23 January 1749, TNA, SP 91/49, fol. 59v.

76. "Carmichael to Newcastle," February 1749, TNA, SP 91/49, fols. 150-57; 153r.

77. "Carmichael to Newcastle," 5 June 1749, TNA SP 91/50, fols. 9-17, 13v.

78. For an overview of Russia's history with scurvy in the eighteenth century, see Bartlett, "Britain, Russia, and Scurvy."

79. Carpenter, *History of Scurvy*, 173-97.

80. Chaplin, "Earthsickness."

81. On the diagnostic challenge, see Carpenter, *History of Scurvy*, 40–42.

82. Fresh air was a frequent cure, see Chaplin, "Earthsickness," 532–33, 541.

83. Waxell, *American Expedition*, 71, 108, 121–22.

84. On scurvy and melancholy, see Carpenter, *History of Scurvy*, 33–37; Lamb, "Rime of the Ancient Mariner"; Lamb, *Preserving the Self*, 114–31.

85. Waxell, *American Expedition*, 127, 129, 128.

86. Waxell, *American Expedition*, 137, 141, 142.

87. Gmelin, *Voyage en Sibérie*, vol. 1:364, 1:365–67.

88. Steller, *Steller's History of Kamchatka*, 227, 274.

89. Steller, *Journal of a Voyage with Bering*, 77, 89, 93.

90. Steller, *Journal of a Voyage with Bering*, 156–57.

91. Waxell, *American Expedition*, 199.

92. Lind, *Treatise of the Scurvy*, 41–42.

93. Lind, *Treatise of Scurvy*, 335–36, 336–37, 337–38.

94. Lind, *Treatise of the Scurvy*, 338–39.

95. Cook, *Voyages and Travels*, 2:609–10, 2:531.

96. Cook, *Voyages and Travels*, 2:38.

97. See Crellin, "Early Settlements in Newfoundland"; Charters, "Disease, Wilderness, Warfare."

98. von Manstein, *Contemporary Memoirs of Russia*, 171.

99. *Florinova ekonomiia*, 339–40. I thank Clare Griffin for this reference.

100. Krafft, *Description et representation*, A2; see also Herzberg, "Nature of Cold," 53–59.

101. "Mr. Miller's letter on incouragement of agriculture, May 17, 1760," RSA, PR/GE/110/9/7.

4. Improving Health, Inoculating Smallpox

1. The academy's results were published in London; see Himsel, "Account of Artificial Cold."

2. Strahlenberg, *Historico-Geographical Description*, 436.

3. Among the works on this topic, see Blum, *Strength in Numbers*; and Cody, *Birthing the Nation*.

4. On the efforts to increase the birth rate, see Kuxhausen, *From the Womb to the Body Politic*.

5. John Alexander focuses on Catherine's government in terms of its intervention to preserve population. In this chapter, I see Catherine's public health policies as an extension of ongoing changes since the 1740s. See Alexander, "Catherine the Great and Public Health."

6. For a discussion of climate determinism in Russia, see Herzberg, "Climate Ideas," 20–24.

7. Montesquieu, *Spirit of Laws*, particularly chaps. 14–17. For a brief discussion of his views of Russia, see Okenfuss, "Catherine, Montesquieu, and Empire," 322–29; and Herzberg, "Climate Ideas," 20–24.

8. All translations are from Montesquieu, *Spirit of Laws*, 1:317–18.

9. Montesquieu, *Spirit of Laws*, 319.

10. Montesquieu, *Spirit of Laws*, 326–27.

11. It was first published as Rulhière, *Anecdotes sur la revolution*, in 1762; and translated into English as *Anecdotes of the Revolution* in 1797.

12. Rulhière, *History or Anecdotes of the Revolution*, 32, 79.

13. Chappe d'Auteroche, *Journey into Siberia*.

14. For example, Chappe d'Auteroche, *Journey into Siberia*, 158–60, which references all the previous authors in assessing Siberia's geography.

15. Chappe d'Auteroche, *Journey into Siberia*, 349.

16. Chappe d'Auteroche, *Journey into Siberia*, 350, 37.

17. Chappe d'Auteroche, *Journey into Siberia*, 353, 351, 351–52.

18. Chappe d'Auteroche, *Journey into Siberia*, 57, 54, 68.

19. Dunlap, "Problem of Syphilitic Children"; Winston, "Medicine, Marriage, and Human Degeneration."

20. The response to his text was the anonymously published *Antidote ou Réfutation*. For a discussion of the Russian reaction to this text, see Levitt, "Antidote to Nervous Juice."

21. "Catherine to Voltaire, 23 January/3 February 1771," in Lentin, *Voltaire and Catherine the Great*, no. 58, 97.

22. "Voltaire to Catherine, 10 July 1771," in Lentin, *Voltaire and Catherine*, no. 70, 111.

23. Romaniello, *Enterprising Empires*, esp. chap. 4.

24. "Macartney to Grafton," 11/22 February 1766, TNA, SP 91/77, fols. 25–34, 25r.

25. "Macartney to Grafton," 11/22 February 1766, TNA, SP 91/77, fols. 25–34, 32v–33r.

26. "Shirley to Weymouth," 28 February/10 March 1768, TNA, SP 91/79, fols. 97–101, 97r–v.

27. "Shirley to Weymouth," 28 February/10 March 1768, TNA, SP 91/79, fols. 97–101, 100v.

28. *PSZ*, vol. 9, no. 6852, 24 December 1735, 662–82.

29. *PSZ*, vol. 9, no. 6852, 24 December 1735, 668.

30. "Claudius Rondeau to Secretary Townshend," 18 May 1730, TNA, SP 91/11, fols. 111–12.

31. Another Scottish physician in Russia, Dr. John Cook, was friendly with L'Estocq throughout the decade. See Cook, *Voyages and Travels*, 2:555–60.

32. Kuxhausen, *From the Womb to the Body*, 33–54.

33. Reichardt produced "De uturi connexione cum mammis," and Lindemann "De partu praeternaturali, quem sine matris aut foetus sectione absolvere non licet operatori."

34. Epatko, "James Mounsey," 7–9.

35. Appleby, "'Rhubarb' Mounsey," 139.

36. Thomas, "Some Correspondence of Dr. James Mounsey," 12–13.

37. For the Royal Society for Arts, Manufactures, and Commerce, see "Letter by Dr. Daniel Dumaresq," 12 July 1760, RSA, PR/GE/110/9/24. For the Royal Society, see Mounsey, "Part of a Letter"; Mounsey, "Strange Effects"; and Weymarn, "Account of an Earthquake."

38. For a contemporary discussion, see "Letter from James Inglis," 22 November 1769, RSA, PR/GE/110/26/110; and "Letter from James Inglis," 11 April 1770, RSA, PR/GE/110/27/140. For a historical assessment, see Appleby, "'Rhubarb' Mounsey"; and Romaniello, "Could Siberian 'Natural Curiosities' Be Replaced?," 260–64.

39. Mounsey and Baker, "Abstract of the Remarkable Case."

40. Mounsey and Baker, "Abstract of the Remarkable Case," 134–35.

41. Mounsey and Baker, "Abstract of the Remarkable Case," 137.

42. Cross, "Chaplains to the British Factory," 130–22; Appleby, "Daniel Dumaresq," 41. The British government received the request for Dumaresq's service to the Russian government early in 1766. See "Letter to Ambassador Vorontsov," 22 April 1766, TNA, SP 100/54.

43. Dumaresq, "Account of that Part of America."

44. *PSZ*, vol. 17, no. 12,785, November 16, 1766, 1050–62.

45. *Ukazy vsepresteleishei*, 111–16.

46. Grombakh, *Russkaia meditsinskaia literatura*, 273–74.

47. "Letter from James Mounsey," 18 June 1762, NRS, GD24/1/846.

48. Timonius, "Account, or History, of the Procuring," 72–73.

49. For an overview, see Miller, *Adoption of Inoculation*, 70–79.

50. On the problems diffusing variolation, see Arnold, "Smallpox and Colonial Medicine"; and Bennett, "Smallpox and Cowpox."

51. Vigor, *Eleven Additional Letters*, 29–30.

52. Bennett, *War Against Smallpox*, 34–35.

53. See a contemporary defense for the value of inoculation, Gilchrist, "Answer to the Objection Against Inoculation."

54. The entire treatment is outlined by Sutton in a letter in John Hope's files in Edinburgh; see "Sutton's directions to one of his pupils," NRS, GD253/143/11/2, fol. 1-12.

55. Weightman, *Great Inoculator*, 59–60.

56. Weightman, *Great Inoculator*, 66–67.

57. Bennett, *War Against Smallpox*, 36–43; Miller, *Adoption of Inoculation*, 237.

58. Clendenning, "Dr. Thomas Dimsdale"; Bartlett, "Russia in the Eighteenth-Century"; Dimsdale, "Mixed Blessing."

59. "Shirley to Weymouth," 6/17 May 1768, TNA, SP 91/79, fols. 117–18, 117v.

60. "Shirley to Weymouth," 17/28 May 1768, TNA, SP 91/79, fol. 119.

61. Dimsdale, *Tracts on Inoculation*, 3.

62. Dimsdale, *Tracts on Inoculation*, 4, 7–8.

63. Dimsdale, *Tracts on Inoculation*, 17–18.

64. "Cathcart to Weymouth," 5/16 September 1768, TNA, SP 91/79, fols. 206–7.

65. Dimsdale, *Tracts on Inoculation*, 19. Schulenius was likely Martin Staehelin (or Shtelin in Russian), who was born 1729 in Riga and died 1792. He completed his medical doctorate at Jena in 1758 with a "Thesis exhibens nonnulas de inflammationebus, in genere consideratis." Shtrenge (Strénge) Andrei Khristian, born Prussia, moved to Russia in 1763; doc med "De inflammatione parium, tam solidarum quam fluidarum in corpore humano" (Erfurt, 1768).

66. Tooke, *View of the Russian Empire*, 1:589.

67. Dimsdate, *Tracts on Inoculation*, 20–21, 23.

68. Dimsdale, *Tracts on Inoculation*, 27–30.

69. Dimsdale, *Tracts on Inoculation*, 27–30.

70. Dimsdale, *Tracts on Inoculation*, 33–34.

71. "Cathcart to Weymouth," 17/28 October 1768, TNA, SP 91/79, fols. 290–92, 290v.

72. There was a debate about the consequence on the bania on inoculation; see Bartlett, "Russia in the Eighteenth-Century," 198–200.

73. Dimsdale, *Tracts on Inoculation*, 35–37.

74. Dimsdale, *Tracts on Inoculation*, 38–40.

75. "Cathcart to Weymouth," 7/18 October 1768, TNA, SP 91/79, fols. 258–61.

76. "Cathcart to Weymouth," 21 October/1 November 1768, TNA, SP 91/79, fols. 293–94, 293v.

77. "Catherine to Voltaire," 6/17 December 1768, in Lentin, *Voltaire and Catherine*, no. 18, 53–54.

78. Voltaire, *Letters Concerning the English*, 73-82.

79. Enish, *Izvestiia o nailuchshem sposobe.*

80. *PSZ*, vol. 19, no. 13,445, 30 March 1770, 47–52

81. Dimsdal', *Nyneshnii sposob privivat' ospy*; *Kratkoe i iasnoe nastavlenie*. For a discussion of the triumph of Dimsdale's method in Russia, see also Alexander, "Communicable Disease," 194–95.

82. Dimsdale, *Tracts on Inoculation*, 102–3, 103.

83. "Opisanie i nastavlenie privivanii ospy."

84. Coxe, *Account of the Prisons and Hospitals*, 20.

85. Bentham Papers, BL, Add MS 33,552, 244v.

86. *PSZ*, vol. 20, no. 14,695, 12 January 1778, 587–88.

87. The official state instruction to Irkutsk is *PSZ*, vol. 19, no. 13,755, 1 February 1772, 444–46; for the remainder, see Tooke, *View of the Russian Empire*,

1:591. The spread of smallpox hospitals is briefly discussed in Bartlett, "Russia in the Eighteenth-Century," 196–97.

88. "Cathcart to Weymouth," 1/12 November 1768, TNA, SP 91/79, fols. 300–11, 302r.

89. Dimsdale, *Tracts on Inoculation*, 118–20.

90. "Letters Patent of Baronage," 13 February 1769, WL, MS 9189/1, fols. 1–2.

91. "Letters Patent of Baronage," 13 February 1769, WL, MS 9189/1, fols. 2–3.

5. Surviving Plague, Mixing Races

1. "Cathcart to Halifax," 24 May/4 June 1771, TNA, SP 91/87, fol. 259–62, 261v.

2. "Cathcart to Halifax," 27 May/7 June 1771, TNA, SP 91/87, fol. 263–65, 264v–265r.

3. On the outbreak of the plague, see Alexander, *Bubonic Plague*, 101–24.

4. Mertens, *Account of the Plague*.

5. "Cathcart to Halifax," 1/12 April 1771, TNA, SP 91/87, fol. 167–69.

6. "Cathcart to Halifax," 5/16 April 1771, TNA, SP 91/87, fol. 170–77, 170r.

7. "Cathcart to Halifax," 28 June/9 July 1771, TNA, SP 91/88, fol. 49–52, 49r–v.

8. "Cathcart to Halifax," 1/12 July 1771, TNA, SP 91/88, fol. 53–55, 53r.

9. "Cathcart to Suffolk," 5/16 July 1771, TNA, SP 91/88, fol. 58–62, 58r.

10. "Cathcart to Suffolk," 8/19 July 1771, TNA, SP 91/88, fol. 65–67, 65r–v.

11. "Cathcart to Suffolk," 12/23 July 1771, TNA, SP 91/88, fol. 68–72, 68r and 71v.

12. "Cathcart to Suffolk," 15/26 July 1771, TNA, SP 91/88, fol. 73–74, 73r.

13. "Cathcart to Suffolk," 26 July/6 August 1771, TNA, SP 91/88, fol. 81–84, 81r.

14. "Cathcart to Suffolk," 12/23 July 1771, TNA, SP 91/88, fol. 68–72, 68r.

15. "Cathcart to Suffolk," 19/20 July 1771, TNA, SP 91/88, fol. 75–78, 75r.

16. "Cathcart to Suffolk," 2/13 August 1771, TNA, SP 91/88, fol. 89–93.

17. Mertens, *Account of the Plague*, 14.

18. Sydenham, *Whole Works*, 5–6.

19. Mertens, *Account of the Plague*, 15.

20. "Cathcart to Suffolk," 26 August/6 September 1771, TNA, SP 91/88, fol. 117–20, 120r–v.

21. "Cathcart to Suffolk," 20 September/1 October 1771, TNA, SP 91/88, fol. 157–59, 157r.

22. "Cathcart to Suffolk," 20 September/1 October 1771, TNA, SP 91/88, fol. 157–59, 157r–v.

23. "Declaration of Count Orloff, Her Imperial Majesty's Adjutant General and Master of the Ordnance," TNA, SP 91/88, fol. 209–210.

24. For a detailed account from Russian sources, see Alexander, *Bubonic Plague*, 177–228; and Kowal, "Danilo Samoilowitz," 434–46.

25. "Cathcart to Suffolk," 27 September/8 October 1771, TNA, SP 91/88, fol. 175–78, 175r–176r.

26. "Cathcart to Suffolk," 27 September/8 October 1771, TNA, SP 91/88, fol. 175–78, 177r.

27. "Cathcart to Suffolk," 4/13 October 1771, TNA, SP 91/88, fol. 202–6.

28. "Cathcart to Suffolk," 11/22 October 1771, TNA, SP 91/88, fols. 207–8, 207r.

29. "Catherine to Voltaire," 6/17 October 1771, in Lentin, *Voltaire and Catherine*, no. 79, 121–22.

30. "Cathcart to Suffolk," 22 November/3 December 1771, TNA, SP 91/88, fols. 260–63, 260r–261r.

31. "Cathcart to Suffolk," 30 December 1771/10 January 1772, TNA, SP 91/89, fol. 21–27, 21r–v.

32. "Cathcart to Suffolk," 30 December 1771/10 January 1772, TNA, SP 91/89, fol. 21–27, 22r.

33. "Ukase or Edict of Her Imperial Majesty, Sovereign of all the Russians from the directing Senate," issued 19 January 1772, TNA, SP 91/89, fol. 103–04.

34. "Recette de la Poudre de fumigation contre la Peste inventeé par la Commission a Moscou, 1771," TNA, SP 91/89, fol. 162–66.

35. "Cathcart to Suffolk," 16/27 March 1772, TNA, SP 91/89, fol. 159–61, 159r.

36. "Ukase, printed at the Senate on 18 March 1772," TNA, SP 91/89, fol. 198–99.

37. "Cathcart to Suffolk," 17/28 April 1772, TNA, SP 91/89, fol. 194–95, 194r.

38. Jones, *Empire of Extinction*, 111–19. On Pallas's later career in Russia, see Jones, "Peter Simon Pallas."

39. Peter Simon Pallas originally published in three volumes in German, between 1771 and 1776. He later published a complete record of all of his travels across the empire in French, *Voyages de M. P. S. Pallas*, in 5 volumes between 1788 and 1793. Johann Gottlieb Georgi published his account in German in 1775, which was translated into English, as *Russia: or, a compleat historical account*.

40. Cross, "Chaplains to the British Factory," 125–42.

41. Skott, "Human Taxonomies," 218–19.

42. The section begins in Georgi, *Russia*, 3:45.

43. Georgi, *Russia*, 1:7–8, 1:23, 1:23–24, 1:22–23.

44. Georgi, *Russia*, 1:35–36 and 45, 1:54, 1:70, 1:95, 2:228.

45. Georgi, *Russia*, 1:117, 2:88, 3:24.

46. Georgi, *Russia*, 2:39, 2:43–44.

47. Georgi, *Russia*, 1:178; 1:191; 3:297, 1:191, 3:297.

48. Georgi, *Russia*, 2:115, 4:22, 4:39, 2:145.

49. Georgi, *Russia*, 3:78, 3:80, 3:116.

50. Georgi, *Russia*, 3:132–33, 3:158, 3:158–59.

51. Georgi, *Russia*, 4:132, 3:151–52.

52. Pallas, *Voyages de M. P. S. Pallas*, 1:499, 1:629.

53. On the importance of racialized bodies, see Curran, *Anatomy of Blackness*; Block, *Colonial Complexions*; Seth, *Difference and Disease*; among others.

54. "Richard Oakes to William Eden," 3/14 January 1777, TNA, SP 91/101, fol. 7–9.

55. Marbault, *Essai sur le commerce*, 28–29.

56. Venechanskii, *Sposoby i nastavleniia*; it was reprinted in Moscow in 1802.

57. Venechanskii, *Sposoby i nastavleniia*, 10.

58. Bakherakht, *O neumerennosti*. See the discussion in Kuxhausen, *From the Womb to the Body Politic*, 18, 88–9.

59. Weisser, "Treating the Secret Disease," 685–86.

60. Coxe, *Account of the Prisons*, 14–15, 15–16.

61. Coxe, *Account of the Prisons*, 14–15, 15.

62. Coxe, *Account of the Prisons*, 23.

63. For his bibliographic details, see Papmehl, "Matthew Guthrie"; and Appleby, "St. Petersburg to Edinburgh."

64. Guthrie, "Medical News."

65. Guthrie, "Part of a Letter," 623.

66. Guthrie, "Part of a Letter," 626–34, 634–35, 635, 636.

67. Mertens, "Observations on the Scurvy," 668–69, 667–8.

68. King, "Letter to the Right Reverend," 7.

69. King, "Letter to the Right Reverend," 9, 11, 22.

70. Guthrie, "Account of the Manner," 328–29, 331.

71. "Samuel to Jeremy Bentham," 8 April 1780, BL, Add. MS 33,557, 188–94, 191–92.

72. "Samuel to Jeremy Bentham," 8 April 1780, BL, Add. MS 33,557, 193.

73. "Samuel to Jeremy Bentham," 19 April 1780, BL, Add. MS 33,557, 196–99, 196.

74. "Samuel to Jeremy Bentham," 19 April 1780, BL, Add. MS 33,557, 198–99.

75. "Samuel to Jeremy Bentham," June 1781, BL, Add. MS 33,557, 301–6, 303.

76. "Harris to Stormont," 17/28 November 1780, TNA, SP 91/106, fol. 182.

77. "Harris to Stormont," 3/14 August 1781, TNA, FO 65/4, no. 113.

78. "Harris to Stormont," 31 August/11 September 1781, TNA, FO 65/4, no. 125.

79. "Harris to Stormont," 21 September/2 October 1781, TNA, FO 65/4, no. 138.

80. "Harris to Stormont," 28 September/9 October 1781, TNA, FO 65/4, no. 141.

81. Cross, *English Lady*, 77–78, 78.

6. Analyzing Catarrh, Overcoming Climate

1. Cullen, *Nosology*, 91, 92.

2. See also the nosological categories for catarrhs in Duncan, *Heads of Lectures*, 163–64.

3. Gagliardi, *Parere sopra l'influenza catarrale*; Sassi, *Due lettere filosofiche Intorno alla Catarrale Influenza*.

4. Mudge, *Radical and Expeditious Cure*, 85–88, 4, 1–2.

5. "Letter from Samuel Bentham to Jeremy Betham," October 20/31, 1781 BL, Add. MS 33,557, fol. 318–24.

6. Bentham Papers, BL, Add. MS 33,552, 111r–v.

7. "Harris to Murray," 24 December 1781/4 January 1782, TNA, FO 65/6, no. 189 (of 1781).

8. "Harris to Murray," 21 January/1 February 1782, TNA, FO 65/6, no. 8 (of 1782).

9. "Harris to Murray," 28 January/8 February 1782, TNA, FO 65/6, no. 9 (of 1782).

10. "Harris to Murray," 4/15 February 1782, TNA, FO 65/6, no. 11 (of 1782).

11. Metzger, *Beytrag zu Geschichte*, 38–39, 40.

12. "Extrait des prima mensis," 170, 172, 173–74.

13. Gunther, "Edward Whitaker Gray."

14. Gray, "Account of the Epidemic Catarrh," 2, 3–4.

15. Toropitsyn, "Vliiane karantinnykh meropriiatii."

16. Gray, "Account of the Epidemic Catarrh," 4.

17. Gray, "Account of the Epidemic Catarrh," 14, 18–19, 22.

18. Gray, "Account of the Epidemic Catarrh," 45–46, 62.

19. Mertens, *Observationes medicae.*

20. Mertens, *Observationes medicae*, 2:34–35, 2:35.

21. Mertens, *Observationes medicae*, 2:38–39, 2:46.

22. "Harris to Grantham," 19/30 September 1782, BA, L29/559/21. His health complaints continued throughout the fall. See also "Harris to Grantham," 1/12 November 1782, BA, L29/559/34; "Harris to Grantham," 6/17 December 1782, BA, L29/559/39/1.

23. For example, Mouritz, *"Flu": A Brief History of Influenza*, 9.

24. Guthrie, *Nouvelles experiences.*

25. Guthrie, "Letter to Dr. Duncan," 367–73.

26. Guthrie, "Letter from Dr. Matthew Guthrie," 328–29.

27. Lesseps, *Travels in Kamtschatka,* 128–29.

28. Guthrie, "Dissertation on the Climate," 214, 215, 222.

29. Guthrie, "Dissertation on the Climate," 225, 226.

30. Guthrie, "Dissertation on the Climate," 218–219, 220, 230.

31. "Rainfall/Precipitation in Saint Petersburg, Russia," Climate.top, accessed December 21, 2020, http://www.saint-petersburg.climatemps.com/precipitation.php.

32. Mertens, *Observationes medicae*, 2:131–32.

33. Mertens, *Observationes medicae*, 2:84, 2:86, 2:93, 2:96.

34. For Tooke's career, see Cross, "Reverend William Tooke's Contribution," 106–15.

35. Tooke, *View of the Russian Empire*, 1:21–22.

36. Tooke, *View of the Russian Empire*, 2:1, 1:21.

37. "Stormont to Harris," 14 January 1780, TNA, SP 91/104, fol. 6–7.

38. "Admiralty to Stormont," 31 January 1780, TNA, SP 91/104, fol. 12.

39. "Stormont to Harris," 11 April 1780, TNA, SP 91/104, fol. 209.

40. "Russian Project for opening the Amoor &c., S. and J. Bentham," sent to Lord Carmarthen, TNA, FO, 97/340, fol. 202–7. On his career, see Alekseev, "Joseph Billings."

41. Sauer, *Account of a Geographical and Astronomical Expedition*; Merck, *Siberia and Northwestern America.*

42. "Character and Manners of the Russians," [1787], box 1, folder 8, BRB, George Macartney Papers, Yale University, 3v–4r.

43. Binney, "Writing the Northern Expedition."

44. "Information concerning Mr Billings Expedition to the North East Part of the Russian Empire and the Coast of America," [1796], fols. 212-215, NLS, MS 1075, fols. 212r–v., 213r., 213r–v.

45. Sauer, *Account of a Geographical and Astronomical Expedition*, 40, 41.

46. Sauer, *Account of a Geographical and Astronomical Expedition*, 124.

47. Guthrie, "Medical News," 434-36.

48. Skott, "Human Taxonomies," 218–19.

49. Sauer, *Account of a Geographical and Astronomical Expedition*, 176.

50. Sarytschew, *Account of a Voyage*, 22.

51. Merck, *Siberia and Northwestern America*, 107.

52. Sauer, *Account of a Geographical and Astronomical Expedition*, 208–9. Merck included a longer version; see *Siberia and Northwestern America*, 142.

53. Sauer, *Account of a Geographical and Astronomical Expedition*, 263, 263–64, 271.

54. Merch, *Siberia and Northwestern America*, 136–37.

55. Sarytschew, *Account of a Voyage*, 31.

56. Krusenstern, *Voyage Round the World*, I, 61–69, 78, 100. Vinkovetsky makes this argument in his article, "Circumnavigation, Empire, Modernity," 197–99.

57. Krusenstern, *Voyage Round the World*, 1:12–13, 1:39, 1:191.

58. Krusenstern, *Voyage Round the World*, 1:108–9.

59. Langsdorff, *Voyages and Travels*, 27, 53.

60. Langsdorff, *Voyages and Travels*, 94.

61. Langsdorff, *Voyages and Travels*, 96–97, 310.

62. *Noctes Russicae*, BL, Add. MS 14,390, 4v.

63. *Noctes Russicae*, BL, Add. MS. 14,390, 140v.

Epilogue

1. On the business relationship, see "John Rogerson to John Clerk," August 23, 1792, NRS, GD18/5121/1.

2. For Crichton's biography, see Tansey, "Life and Works"; and Appleby, "Sir Alexander Crichton."

3. Crichton, *Inquiry into the Nature and Origin.*

4. Tansey, "Life and Works," 248.

5. Crichton et al., *Russische Sammlung.*

6. Beddoes, *Observations on the Nature and Cure.*

7. Beddoes, "Observations on the nature," 67–86.

8. Beddoes, "Observations on the nature," 68.

9. Beddoes, "Observations on the nature," 85.

10. Crichton, *Account of Some Experiments*, 10.

11. N.'s case is recorded in Crichton, *Account of Some Experiments*, 11–15.

12. Beddoes, "Observations on the nature," 79–80.

13. Crichton, *Account of Some Experiments*, 15–18.

14. Crichton, *Account of Some Experiments*, 18–19, 46.

15. Crichton, *Practical Observations*, xxix, xxix–xxx.
16. Crichton, *Practical Observations*, 50–51, 52, 21, 52.
17. Tansey, "Life and Works," 251, 253.
18. Mauricheau-Beaupré, *Treatise on the Effects*, xvii–xviii, 82, 83.
19. Mauricheau-Beaupré, *Treatise on the Effects*, 93.
20. Larrey, *Surgical Memoirs*, 81, 80.

Bibliography

Archival Sources

Bedfordshire Archives, Bedford, Great Britain

L 29/559, Correspondence between Thomas Robinson 2nd Baron Grantham (1738–1786) as Foreign Secretary and Sir James Harris, Ambassador at St. Petersburg

Beinecke Rare Book and Manuscript Library, Yale University, New Haven, CT

George Macartney Papers

The British Library, Manuscripts, London

Add. MS 14,390, *Noctes Russicae, or Russian evening recreations*
Bentham Papers, Add. MS 33,552, 33,557
Blenheim Papers, Add. MS 61149
Hans Sloane MS 3237, 4054, 4055, 4056
Tyrawley Papers, Add. MS 23361

Library Carolina Rediviva, University of Uppsala, Sweden

Linnaean correspondence

The National Archives, Kew, Richmond, Surrey, Great Britain

CO 389, Board of Trade: Entry Books
FO 65, Foreign Office: General correspondence before 1906, Russian Empire
FO 97/340, Russia: Letters and Papers, supplementary
SP 91, State Papers Foreign: Russia
SP 100/54, Foreign Ministers in England, Russia

National Library of Scotland, Special Collections, Edinburgh

MS 1075, Melville Papers
MS 5163, Paul Papers

National Records of Scotland, Edinburgh

GD1/42/1, Papers of the Family of Aytoun of Inchdernie, Fife
GD24, Papers of the Family Stirling Home Dummond Moray of Abercairny
GD253/143, Medical Papers of John Hope MD
GD253/145, Botanical Papers of John Hope MD

Royal Society for Arts Archive, London

PR/GE/110/9/7, "Mr. Miller's letter on incouragement of agriculture"
PR/GE/110/9/15, "Letter from D. Wolfe about Polish manna"
PR/GE/110/9/24, "Letter by Dr. Daniel Dumaresq"
PR/GE/110/26/110, "Letter from James Inglis"
PR/GE/110/27/140, "Letter from James Inglis"

Wellcome Library, Rare Materials, London

MS 1143, J. F. Bernard, *A Relation of Grand Tartary, drawn up from the Original Memoirs of the Suedes, who were Prisoners in Siberia, during the War between Sueden and Russia*, translated by William Farrington
MS 9189, Baron Thomas Dimsdale (1712–1800)

Published Primary Sources

Allison, Thomas. *An Account of a Voyage from Archangel in Russia in the Year 1697*. London: D. Brown, 1699.
Alston, Charles. "A Dissertation on the Sexes of Plants." In *Essays and Observation, Physical and Literary*, vol. 1, 205–83. Edinburgh: G. Hamilton and J. Balfour, 1754.
Amman, Johann. *Stirpium Rariorum in Imperio Rutheno Sponte Provenientium Icones et Descriptiones*. St. Petersburg, 1739.
Avril, Philippe. *Travels Into divers Parts of Europe and Asia*. London, 1693.
Bakherakht, A. G. *O neumerennosti v liubostrastii oboikh polov*. St. Petersburg, 1779.
"Beddoes, Thomas, M.D. Observations on the nature and cure of Calculus, Sea Scurvy, Consumption, Catarrh, and Fever; Together with Conjectures Upon Several Other Subjects of Physiology and Pathology." In *Medical and Commentaries for the Year 1793*, vol. 8, 67–86. Edinburgh: Peter Hill, 1794.
Beddoes, Thomas. *Observations on the Nature and Cure of Calculus, Sea Scurvy, Consumption, Catarrh, and Fever*. London: J. Murray, 1793.
Bell, John. *Travels from St. Petersburg in Russia to Divers Parts of Asia*. 2 vols. Glasgow: John Bell and Robert and Andrew Foulis, 1763.
Bentham, Jeremy. *A Fragment on Government*. Oxford: Clarendon Press, 1891.
Bernard, J. F. *Recueil du voyages au Nord*. 10 vols. Amsterdam, 1715–1738.

Birch, Thomas, ed. *A Collection of the State Papers of John Thurloe, Esq.* 7 vols. London, 1742.

Boyle, Robert. *New Experiments and Observations Touching Cold.* London: John Crook, 1665.

Brand, Adam. *A Journal of the Embassy from Their Majesties John and Peter Alexievitz, Emperors of Muscovy, &c. Over Land into China.* London, 1698.

Breyne, John Philip. "A letter from John Phil. Breyne, M.D. F.R.S. to Sir Hans Sloane, Bart. Pres. R. S. with Observations, and a Description of Some Mammoth's Bones Dug up in Siberia, Proving Them to Have Belonged to Elephants." *Philosophical Transactions of the Royal Society of London* 40 (1738): 124–38.

Chappe d'Auteroche, Jean-Baptiste. *A Journey into Siberia, Made by Order of the King of France.* London: T. Jeffreys, 1770.

Collins, Samuel. *The Present State of Russia.* London: John Winter, 1671.

Cook, John. *Voyages and Travels through the Russian Empire, Tartary, and Part of the Kingdom of Persia.* 2 vols. Edinburgh, 1770.

Coxe, William. *Account of the Prisons and Hospitals in Russia, Sweden, and Denmark with Occasional Remarks on the Different Modes of Punishment in Those Countries.* London: T. Cadell, 1781.

Crichton, Alexander. *An Account of Some Experiments made with the Vapour of Boiling Tar, in the Cure of Pulmonary Consumption.* Edinburgh: James Ballantyne, 1817.

Crichton, Alexander. *An Inquiry into the Nature and Origin of Mental Derangement. Comprehending a Concise System of the Physiology and Pathology of the Human Mind, and a History of the Passions and Their Effects.* 2 vols. London: T. Cadell and W. Davies, 1798.

Crichton, Alexander. *Practical Observations on the Treatment and Cure of Several Varieties of Pulmonary Consumption, and on the Vapour of Boiling Tar in That Disease.* London: Lloyd and Son, 1823.

Crichton, Alexander, Joseph Rehmann, and Karl Friedrich Burdach. *Russische Sammlung für Naturwissenschaft und Heilkunst.* 1815.

Cross, A. G., ed. *An English Lady at the Court of Catherine the Great: The Journal of Baroness Elizabeth Dimsdale, 1781.* Cambridge, UK: Crest, 1989.

Crull, Jodocus. *An Account of the Antient and Present State of Muscovy.* 2 vols. London: A. Roper and A. Bosvile, 1698.

Cullen, William. *Nosology: Or, A Systematic Arrangement of Diseases, by Classes, Orders, Genera, and Species.* Edinburgh: C. Stewart, 1800.

Dale, Samuel. *Pharmacologiae, seu Manductionis and Materiam Medicam Supplementum.* London: Sam. Smith and Benj. Walford, 1705.

Dimsdal', T. *Kratkoe i iasnoe nastavlenie kakim obrazom soderzhat' bol'nogo . . . v ospe po metody gospodina barona Dimsdalia.* St. Petersburg, 1770.

Dimsdal', T. *Nyneshnii sposob privivat' ospy (perevod s angliiskogo L. Sichkareva).* St. Petersburg, 1770.

Dimsdale, Thomas. *Tracts on Inoculation.* London: James Philipps, 1781.

Dixon, Simon, ed. *Britain and Russia in the Age of Peter the Great: Historical Documents.* London: School of Slavonic and East European Studies, 1998.

Dumaresq, Daniel. "An Account of that Part of America, which is nearest to the Land of Kamtchatka." *Philosophical Transactions of the Royal Society of London* 51 (1759): 477–97.

Duncan, Andrew. *Heads of Lectures on the Theory and Practice of Medicine*. 2nd ed. Edinburgh: C. Eliot, 1781.

Enish, I. G. *Izvestiia o nailuchshem sposobe dlia privivaniia ospy (perevod s nemetskogo I. B.)*. St. Petersburg, 1769.

Euler, Leonard. "Extract of a Letter from Mr. Leonard Euler, Prof. Mathem. And Member of the Imperial Society at St. Petersburgh, to the Rev. Mr. Cha. Westein, Chaplain and Secretary to His Royal Highness the Prince of Wales, concerning the Discoveries of the Russians on the North-East Coast of Asia." *Philosophical Transactions of the Royal Society of London* 44 (1747): 421–23.

"Extrait des prima mensis de la faculté de médecine de Paris, tenus les 15 juin & 4 juillet 1782." *Journal de Médecine, Chirugie, Pharmacie, &c.* 58 (July 1782): 170–84.

Fletcher, Giles. *Of the Russe Common Wealth, Or Maner of Government by the Russe Emperour (commonly called the Emperour of Muskovia (with the manners, and fashions of the people of that Countrey)*. London: Thomas Charde, 1591.

Florinova ekonomiia v deviati knigakh sostoiashchaia. St. Petersburg: Imperatorskii akademii nauk, 1760.

Fothergill, John. "An Account of the Some Observations and Experiments made in Siberia, extracted from the Preface to the *Flora Sibirica*." *Philosophical Transactions of the Royal Society of London* 45 (1748): 248–62.

Gagliardi, Domenico. *Parere sopra l'influenza catarrale, che presentemente regna in Roma, e Stato Ecclesiastico*. Rome: Reuerenda Camera Apostolica, 1730.

Gal'perin, S. A., and I. R. Tarkhanov. *Angliiskaia boliezn' rakhit*. St. Petersburg: Tipografiia Tov-va "Narodnaia pol'za." 1899.

Georgi, Johann Gottlieb. *Russia: or, a compleat historical account of all the nations which compose that empire*. 4 vols. Translated by William Tooke. London, 1780–1783.

Gilchrist, Ebenezer. "Answer to the Objection against Inoculation." In *Essays and Observations, Physical and Literary*, vol. 2, 396–402. Edinburgh: G. Hamilton and J. Balfour, 1756.

Gmelin, Johann Georg. *Reise durch Sibirien von dem Jahr 1733 bis 1734*. 4 vols. Göttingen: Verlegts Abram Vandenhoeckss eel. Wittwe, 1751–1752.

Gmelin, Johann Georg. *Voyage en Sibérie*. 2 vols. Paris: Desaint, 1767.

Gray, Edward. "An Account of the Epidemic Catarrh, of the year 1782, compiled at the request of the Society." *Medical Communications* 1 (London: Joseph Johnson, 1784): 1–70.

Guthrie, Matthew. "Account of the Manner in which the Russians treat Persons affected by the Fumes of burning Charcoal, and other Effluvia of the same Nature." *Philosophical Transactions of the Royal Society of London* 69 (1779): 325–31.

Guthrie, Matthew. "A Dissertation on the Climate of Russia." *Transactions of the Royal Society of Edinburgh* 2 (1790): 213–33.

Guthrie, Matthew. "A Letter from Dr. Matthew Guthrie Physician at St. Petersburgh, to Dr Duncan, on the Effects of a cold Climate on the Land Scurvy, &c." *Medical Commentaries for the Year 1787* 22 (1788): 328–29.

Guthrie, Matthew. "A Letter to Dr. Duncan from Matthew Guthrie." *Medical Commentaries for the Year 1785* 20 (1786): 367–73.

Guthrie, Matthew. "Medical News." *Medical and Philosophical Commentaries* 5, part 1 (1777): 434–36.

Guthrie, Matthew. "Part of a Letter from Matthew Guthrie, M.D. of Petersburgh, to Dr. Priestly, F.R.S. on the Regimen of the Natives of Russia." *Philosophical Transactions of the Royal Society of London* 68 (1778): 622–36.

Guthrie, Matthew. *Nouvelles experiences pour servir à determiner le vrai point de congelation du mercure.* St. Petersburg, 1785.

Himsel, Dr. "An Account of Artificial Cold produced at St. Peterburg." *Philosophical Transactions of the Royal Society of London* 51 (1759): 670–76.

Ides, E. Ysbrant. *Three Years Travels from Moscow over-land to China.* London, 1705.

Johnson, J. *A Guide for Gentlemen Studying Medicine at the University of Edinburgh.* London: G. G. J. and J. Robinson, 1792.

King, John Glen. "A Letter to the Right Reverend The Lord Bishop of Durham, Containing Some Observations on the Climate of Russia, and the Northern Countries." London: J. Dodsley, 1778.

Krafft, George Wolffgang. *Description et representation exacte de la maison de glace, construite a St. Petersbourg au mois de Janvier 1740.* St. Petersburg: Academy of Sciences, 1741.

Krusenstern, Adam J. von. *Voyage Round the World in the Years 1803, 1804, 1805, and 1806.* Translated by Richard Belgrave Hoppner. 2 vols. London: John Murray, 1813.

Langsdorff, G. H. von. *Voyages and Travels in Various Parts of the World during the Years 1803, 1804, 1805, 1806, and 1807.* London: Henry Colburn, 1814.

Larrey, D. J. *Surgical Memoirs of the Campaigns of Russia, Germany, and France.* Translated by John C. Mercer. Philadelphia: Carey and Lea, 1832.

Lesseps, Jean Baptiste-Bartelemy de. *Travels in Kamtschatka, during the Years 1787 and 1788.* 2 vols. London: J. Johnson, 1790.

Lentin, A., ed. and trans. *Voltaire and Catherine the Great: Selected Correspondence.* Cambridge, MA: Oriental Research Partners, 1974.

Lind, James, *A Treatise of the Scurvy, in Three Parts.* Edinburgh: Sands, Murray, and Cochran, 1753.

L'Isle, Joseph Nicholas de. "Extract of a Letter to the publisher from Mons. De Lisle, Astronomer Royal at Petersburgh, containing his observations of the eclipses of Jupiter's satellites." *Philosophical Transactions of the Royal Society of London* 36 (1729): 37–38.

L'Isle, Jospeh Nicholas de. "A proposal for the measurement of the Earth in Russia." *Philosophical Transactions of the Royal Society of London* 40 (1737): 27–49.

Manstein, C. H. von. *Contemporary Memoirs of Russia from the Year 1727 to 1744.* 2nd ed. New York: Da Capo, 1968.

Marbault. *Essai sur le commerce de Russie, avec l'histoire de ses découvertes.* Amsterdam, 1777.

Mauricheau-Beaupré, Pierre Jean. *A Treatise on the Effects and Properties of Cold.* Translated by John Clendinning. Edinburgh, 1826.

Merck, Carl Heinrich. *Siberia and Northwestern America, 1788–1792: The Journal of Carl Heinrich Merck, Naturalist with the Russian Scientific Expedition Led by Captains Joseph Billings and Gavriil Sarychev.* Translated by Fritz Jaensch. Edited by Richard A. Pierce. Kingston, ON: Limestone, 1980.

Mertens, Charles de. *An Account of the Plague which Raged at Moscow in 1771.* Translated by Richard Pearson. London, 1799.

Mertens, Charles de. *Observationes medicae de febribus, putridis, de peste munn ullisque aliis morbis.* 2 vols. Pavia: Monasterii S. Salvator & B. Cominus, 1791.

Mertens, Charles de. "Observations on the Scurvy." *Philosophical Transactions of the Royal Society of London* 68 (1778): 661-80.

Metzger, J. D. *Beytrag zu Geschichte der Frühlings Epidemie im Zahr 1782.* Königsberg, 1782.

Montesquieu. *The Spirit of Laws.* Translated by Mr. Nugent. London: J. Nourse and P. Vaillant, 1752.

Mounsey, James. "An Account of an Earthquake in Siberia: In a Letter from Mons. Weyman to Dr. Mounsey, Principal Physician of the Emperor of Russia, F.R.S." *Philosophical Transactions of the Royal Society of London* 53 (1763): 201-10.

Mounsey, James. "Part of a Letter from James Mounsey, M.D. Physician to the Czarina's Army, to Mr. Henry Baker, F.R.S. concerning the Russia Castor, the Baths at Carlsbad, the Salt-Mines near Cracau, and Various other Notices." *Philosophical Transactions of the Royal Society of London* 46 (1749): 217-32.

Mounsey, James. "The Strange Effects of Some Effervescent Mixtures; In a Letter from Dr. James Mounsey, Physician to of the Russian Army, and F.R.S. to Mr. Henry Baker, F.R.S." *Philosophical Transactions of the Royal Society of London* 50 (1757): 19-22.

Mounsey, James, and Henry Baker. "An Abstract of the Remarkable Case and Cure of a Woman, from Whom a Foetus Was Extracted, That Had Been Lodged Thirteen Years in One of the Fallopian Tubes." *Philosophical Transactions of the Royal Society of London* 45 (1748): 131-37.

Mouritz, A. *"The Flu": A Brief History of Influenza in U.S. America, Europe, Hawai'i.* Honolulu: Advertiser Publishing, 1921.

Mudge, John. *A Radical and Expeditious Cure for a Recent Catarrhous Cough.* London: E. Allen, 1778.

Muller, John Bernard. "The Manners and Customs of the Ostiacks." In *The Present State of Russia*, vol. 2. London: W. Taylor, 1723.

Okhotina-Lind, Natal'ia, and Peter Ul'f Meller, eds. *Vtoraia kamchatskaia ekspeditsiia: Dokumenty 1734–1736.* St. Petersburg: Nestor-Istoriia, 2009.

Olearius, Adam. *Vermehrte Newe Beschreibung Der Muscowitischen und Persischen Reyse.* Schleswig, 1656.

"Opisanie i nastavlenie privivanii ospy." *Trudy vol'nago ekonomicheskago obshchestva, k pooshchreniiu v Rossii zemledeliia i dom ostroitel'stva.* 21 (1772): 65-116.

Pallas, Peter Simon. *Voyages de M. P. S. Pallas, en différentes provinces de l'empire de Russie, et dans l'Asie septentrionale.* Translated by Gauthier de la Peyronie. 5 vols. Paris: Maradan, 1788-1793.

Polnoe sobranie zakonov Rossiiskoi Imperii (PSZ). Series 1, 45 vols. St. Petersburg: Tipografiia II otdeleniia sobstvennoi ego Imperatorskago Velichestva Kantseliarii, 1830.

Rulhière, Claude-Carloman de. *A History or Anecdotes of the Revolution in Russia in the Year 1762*. London: M. Beauvalet, 1797.

Sarytschew, Gawrila. *Account of a Voyage of Discovery to the North-East of Siberia, the Frozen Ocean, and the North-East Sea*. London: Richard Phillips, 1806.

Sassi, Giuseppe Antonio. *Due lettere filosofiche Intorno alla Catarrale Influenza feguita in quest' anno 1730, universalmente per tutta l'Europa, e per altre parti del Mondo*. Milan: Eredi di Domenico Bellagatta, 1730.

Sauer, Martin. *An Account of a Geographical and Astronomical Expedition to the Northern Parts of Russia*. London, 1802.

[Dr. Skinner]. *Some Observations Made upon the Russia Seed, Shewing Its Admirable Virtues in Curing the Rickets in Children*. London, 1694.

Sloane, Hans. "An account of the elephants teeth and bones found under ground." *Philosophical Transactions of the Royal Society of London* 35 (1728): 457–71.

Smith, James Edward, ed. *A Selection of the Correspondence of Linnaeus and Other Naturalists, From the Original Manuscripts*. 2 vols. London, 1821.

Steller, Georg Wilhelm. *Steller's History of Kamchatka: Collected Information Concerning the History of Kamchatka, Its Peoples, Their Manners, Names, Lifestyle, and Various Customary Practices*. Edited by Marvin W. Falk. Translated by Margritt Engel and Karen Willmore. Fairbanks: University of Alaska Press, 2003.

Steller, George Wilhelm. *Journal of a Voyage with Bering, 1741–1742*. Edited by O. W. Frost. Translated by Margritt A. Engel and O. W. Frost. Stanford, CA: Stanford University Press, 1988.

Strahlenberg, Philip Johan von. *An Historico-Geographical Description of the North and Eastern Parts of Europe and Asia*. London, 1738.

Struys, John. *The Perilous and most Unhappy Voyages of John Struys through Italy, Greece, Lifeland, Moscovia, Tartary, Media, Persia, East-India, Japan, and other Places in Europe, Africa and Asia*. Translated by John Morrison. London: Samuel Smith, 1683.

Sydenham, Thomas. *The Whole Works of that Excellent Practical Physician, Dr. Thomas Sydenham*. 3rd ed. Translated by John Pechy. London: R. Wellington, 1701.

Thomas, Graham C. G. "Some Correspondence of Dr. James Mounsey, Physician to the Empress Elizabeth of Russia." *Scottish Slavonic Review* 4 (1985): 12–13.

Tikhomirov, Grigor'. *Pravila o sposobe vrachevaniia Angliiskoi bolezni*. St. Petersburg: Tip. N. Gracha, 1830.

Timonius, Emanuel. "An Account, or History, of the Procuring of the Small-Pox by Incision, or Inoculation; as it has for some time been practised at Constantinople." *Philosophical Transactions of the Royal Society of London* 29 (1714): 72–82.

Tooke, William. *View of the Russian Empire during the Reign of Catharine the Second and to the Close of the Eighteenth Century*. 2 vols. London: T. H. Longman and O. Rees, 1799.

Ukazy vsepresteleishei Derzhavneshei, Velikoi Gosudaryni imperatritsy Ekateriny Alekseevny samoderzhitsy vserossiiskoi. St. Petersburg: Senat, 1767.

Venechanskii, S. A. *Sposoby i nastavleniia, po kotorym zarazhennye frantsuzskoiu bolezniiu*. St. Petersburg, 1776.

Vigor, Jane. *Eleven Additional Letters from Russia, in the Reign of Peter II*. London: Dodsley, 1785.

Voltaire. *Letters Concerning the English Nation*. London: C. Davis and A. Lyon, 1733.

Watson, William. "An Account of the Treatise, presented to the Royal Society, intitled, *Flora Sibirica, five historia plantarum Sibiriae tomus secundus*." *Philosophical Transactions of the Royal Society of London* 48 (1753): 141–52.

Waxell, Sven. *The American Expedition*. London: William Hodges, 1952.

Weymarn, W. W. "An Account of an Earthquake in Siberia, In a Letter from Mons. Weymarn to Dr. Mounsey, Principal Physician of the Emperor of Russia, F.R.S." *Philosophical Transactions of the Royal Society of London* 53 (1763): 201–10.

Zhukovskii, V. P. *Rakhit: angliiskaia boliezn'*. St. Petersburg: Izdatel'stvo zhurnala "Prakticheskia medtsina," 1897.

Secondary Sources

Afinogenov, Gregory. *Spies and Scholars: Chinese Secrets and Imperial Russia's Quest for World Power*. Cambridge, MA: Harvard University Press, 2020.

Alekseev, A. I. "Joseph Billings." *Geographical Journal* 132, no. 2 (1966): 233–38.

Alexander, John T. *Bubonic Plague in Early Modern Russia: Public Health and Urban Disaster*. New York: Oxford University Press, 2003.

Alexander, John T. "Catherine the Great and Public Health." *Journal of the History of Medicine and Allied Sciences* 36, no. 2 (1981): 185–204.

Alexander, John T. "Communicable Disease, Anti-Epidemic Policies, and the Role of Medical Professionals in Russia, 1725–62." *Canadian-American Slavic Studies* 12, no. 1 (1978): 155–69.

Alexander, John T. "Medical Developments in Petrine Russia." *Canadian-American Slavic Studies* 8, no. 2 (1974): 198–221.

Alimento, Antonella. "Entre 'les moeurs des Crétois et les loix de Minos': la pénétration et la réception du mouvement physiocratique française en Suède (1767–1795)." *Histoire, Économie et Société* 29, no. 1 (2010): 68–80.

Anemone, Anthony. "The Monsters of Peter the Great: The Culture of the St. Petersburg Kunstkamera in the Eighteenth Century." *Slavic and East European Journal* 44, no. 4 (2000): 583–602.

Appleby, Andrew B. "Epidemics and Famines in the Little Ice Age." *Journal of Interdisciplinary History* 10, no. 4 (1980): 643–66.

Appleby, John H. "Daniel Dumaresq, D.D., F.R.S. (1712–1805) as a Promoter of Anglo-Russian Science and Culture." *Notes and Records of the Royal Society of London* 44, no. 1 (1990): 25–50.

Appleby, John H. "The Founding of St. Petersburg in the Context of the Royal Society's Relationship with Russia." *Notes and Records of the Royal Society of London* 57, no. 3 (2003): 273–84.

Appleby, John H. "'Rhubarb' Mounsey and the Surinam Toad: A Scottish Physician-Naturalist in Russia." *Archives of Natural History* 11, no. 1 (1982): 25–50.

Appleby, John H. "St. Petersburg to Edinburgh: Matthew Guthrie's Introduction of Medicinal Plants in the Context of Scottish-Russian Natural History Exchange." *Archives of Natural History* 14, no. 1 (1987): 45–58.

Appleby, John H. "Sir Alexander Crichton, F.R.S. (1763–1856), Imperial Russian Physician at Large." *Notes and Records of the Royal Society of London* 53, no. 2 (1999): 219–30.

Arner, Katherine. "Making Global Commerce into Health Diplomacy: Consuls and Commercial Agents in the Age of Atlantic Revolution." *Journal of World History* 24, no. 4 (2013): 771–96.

Arnold, David. "Introduction: Tropical Medicine before Manson." In *Warm Climates and Western Medicine: The Emergence of Tropical Medicine, 1500–1900*, edited by David Arnold, 1–19. Amsterdam: Rodopoi, 1996.

Arnold, David. "Smallpox and Colonial Medicine in Nineteenth-Century India." In *Imperial Medicine and Indigenous Societies*, edited by David Arnold, 45–65. Manchester: Manchester University Press, 1988.

Archer, Seth. *Sharks Upon the Land: Colonialism, Indigenous Health, and Culture in Hawai'i, 1778–1855*. New York: Cambridge University Press, 2018.

Arrizabalaga, Jon, John Henderson, and Roger French. *The Great Pox: The French Disease in Renaissance Europe*. New Haven, CT: Yale University Press, 1997.

Barca, Manuel. *The Yellow Demon of Fever: Fighting Disease in the Nineteenth-Century Transatlantic Slave Trade*. New Haven, CT: Yale University Press, 2020.

Bartlett, Roger. "Britain, Russia, and Scurvy in the Eighteenth Century." *Oxford Slavonic Papers* 29 (1996): 23–43.

Bartlett, Roger. "Russia in the Eighteenth-Century European Adoption of Inoculation for Smallpox." In *Russia and the World of the Eighteenth Century*, edited by R. P. Bartlett, A. G. Cross, and Karen Rasmussen, 193–213. Columbus, OH: Slavica, 1988.

Bay, Alexander R. *Beriberi in Modern Japan: The Making of a National Disease*. Rochester, NY: University of Rochester Press, 2012.

Behringer, Wolfgang. *A Cultural History of Climate*. Translated by Patrick Camiller. Malden, MA: Polity, 2007.

Belbourgo, James. *Collecting the World: Hans Sloane and the Origins of the British Museum*. Cambridge, MA: Harvard University Press, 2017.

Bennett, Michael J. "Smallpox and Cowpox Under the Southern Cross: The Smallpox Epidemic of 1789 and the Advent of Vaccination in Colonial Australia." *Bulletin of the History of Medicine* 83, no. 1 (2009): 37–62.

Bennett, Michael. *War Against Smallpox: Edward Jenner and the Global Spread of Vaccination*. New York: Cambridge University Press, 2020.

Binney, Matthew W. "Writing the Northern Expedition, 1785–1793: Martin Sauer's *An Account of a Geographical and Astronomical Expedition to the Northern Parts of Russia* (1802)." *Studies in Travel Writing* 22, no. 2 (2018): 121–41.

Birken, William. "The Dissenting Tradition in English Medicine of the Seventeenth and Eighteenth Centuries." *Medical History* 39 (1995): 197–218.

Bishop, W. J. "English Physicians in Russia in the Sixteenth and Seventeenth Centuries." *Proceedings of the Royal Society of Medicine* (1929): 143-52.

Biskup, Thomas. "The University of Göttingen and the Personal Union, 1737-1837." In *The Hanoverian Dimension in British History, 1714–1837*, edited by Brendan Simms and Torsten Riotte, 128-60. New York: Cambridge University Press, 2003.

Black, J. L. "G-.F. Müller and the Russian Academy of Sciences Contingent in the Second Kamchatka Expedition, 1733-1743." *Canadian Slavonic Papers* 25, no. 2 (1983): 235-52.

Black, Lydia T. *Russians in Alaska, 1732–1867*. Anchorage: University of Alaska Press, 2004.

Bleys, Rudy C. *The Geography of Perversion: Male-to-Male Sexual Behavior Outside the West and the Ethnographic Imagination*. New York: New York University Press, 1995.

Block, Sharon. *Colonial Complexions: Race and Bodies in Eighteenth-Century America*. Philadelphia: University of Pennsylvania Press, 2018.

Blum, Carol. *Strength in Numbers: Population, Reproduction, and Power in Eighteenth-Century France*. Baltimore, NJ: Johns Hopkins University Press, 2002.

Bogdanov, A. B. *Materialy dlia biograficheskogo spravochnika russkikh vrachei XVII-XX vv*. St. Petersburg: Evropeiskii universitet v Sankt-Peterburge, 2014.

Bonner, Thomas Neville. *Becoming a Physician: Medical Education in Britain, France, Germany, and the United States, 1750–1945*. New York: Oxford University Press, 1995.

Boterbloem, Kees. *The Fiction and Reality of Jan Struys: A Seventeenth-Century Dutch Globetrotter*. New York: Palgrave, 2008.

Boterbloem, Kees. *Moderniser of Russia: Andrei Vinius, 1641–1716*. New York: Palgrave Macmillan, 2013.

Bowers, Kristy Wilson. *Plague and Public Health in Early Modern Seville*. Rochester, NY: University of Rochester Press, 2013.

Brescius, Moritz von. *German Science in the Age of Empire: Enterprise, Opportunity and the Schlagintweit Brothers*. New York: Cambridge University Press, 2018.

Brikner, A. G. "Chuma v Moskve v 1654 godu." *Istoricheskii vestnik: Istoriko-literaturnyi zhurnal* 16 (April 1884): 5-23.

Broberg, Gunnar. "*Homo Sapiens*: Linnaeus's Classification of Man." In *Linnaeus: The Man and His Work*, edited by Tore Frängsmyr, 156-194. Berkeley: University of California Press, 1983.

Broman, Thomas H. *The Transformation of German Academic Medicine, 1750–1820*. New York: Cambridge University Press, 1996.

Brückner, Alexander. *Die Aerzte in Russland bis zum Jahre 1800*. St. Petersburg, 1887.

Bruijn, Iris. *Ship's Surgeons of the Dutch East India Company: Commerce and the Progress of Medicine in the Eighteenth Century*. Leiden: Leiden University Press, 2009.

Bryce, W. J. "Russian Collections in the Sloane Herbarium." *Archives of Natural History* 32, no. 1 (2005): 26-33.

Burgess, Renate. "Thomas Garvine: Ayrshire Surgeon Active in Russia and China." *Medical History* 19, no. 1 (1975): 91-95.

Butler, Judith. "Foucault and the Paradox of Bodily Inscriptions." *Journal of Philosophy* 86, no. 11 (1989): 601–7.

Cagle, Hugh. *Assembling the Tropics: Science and Medicine in Portugal's Empire, 1450–1700*. New York: Cambridge University Press, 2018.

Cain, A. J. "Logic and Memory in Linnaeus's System of Taxonomy." *Proceedings of the Linnaean Society of London* 169 (1958): 144–63.

Carpenter, Kenneth J. *The History of Scurvy and Vitamin C*. New York: Cambridge University Press, 1986.

Cates, Gerald L. "The 'Seasoning': Disease and Death Among the First Colonist of Georgia." *Georgia Historical Quarterly* 64 (1980): 146–58.

Chakrabarty, Dipesh. *Provincializing Europe: Postcolonial Thought and Historical Difference*. Princeton, NJ: Princeton University Press, 2000.

Chaplin, Joyce E. "Earthsickness: Circumnavigation and the Terrestrial Human Body, 1520–1800." *Bulletin of the History of Medicine* 86, no. 4 (2012): 515–42.

Chaplin, Joyce E. *Subject Matter: Technology, the Body, and Science on the Anglo-American Frontier, 1500–1676*. Cambridge, MA: Harvard University Press, 2001.

Charters, Erica M. "Disease, Wilderness, Warfare, and Imperial Relations: The Battle for Quebec, 1759–1760." *War in History* 16, no. 1 (2009): 1–24.

Chase-Levenson, Alex. *The Yellow Flag: Quarantine and the British Mediterranean World, 1780–1860*. New York: Cambridge University Press, 2020.

Cheek, Pamela. *Sexual Antipodes: Enlightenment Globalization and the Placing of Sex*. Stanford, CA: Stanford University Press, 2003.

Chistovich, Ia. *Istoriia pervykh meditsynskikh shkol v Rossii*. St. Petersburg: Tipografiia Iakov Treia, 1883.

Chrissidis, Nikolaos A. *An Academy at the Court of the Tsars: Greek Scholars and Jesuit Education in Early Modern Russia*. Dekalb: Northern Illinois University Press, 2016.

Clendenning, Philip H. "Dr. Thomas Dimsdale and Smallpox Inoculation in Russia." *Journal of the History of Medicine and Allied Sciences* 28 (1973): 109–25.

Cody, Lisa Forman. *Birthing the Nation: Sex, Science, and the Conception of Eighteenth-Century Britons*. New York: Oxford University Press, 2005.

Cole, Richard G. "In Search of a New Mentality: The Interface of Academic and Popular Medicine in the Sixteenth Century." *Journal of Popular Culture* 26, no. 4 (1993): 155–72.

Cook, Alexandra. "Linnaeus and Chinese Plants: A Test of the Linguistic Imperialism Thesis." *Notes and Records of the Royal Society* 64 (2010): 121–38.

Cook, Harold J. "The History of Medicine and the Scientific Revolution." *Isis* 102, no. 1 (2011): 101–8.

Cook, Harold J. *Matters of Exchange: Commerce, Medicine, and Science in the Dutch Golden Age*. New Haven, CT: Yale University Press, 2007.

Cooper, Alix. *Inventing the Indigenous: Local Knowledge and Natural History in Early Modern Europe*. New York: Cambridge University Press, 2007.

Craig, Stephen C. "'Enquire into All the Circumstances of the Patient Narrowly': John Rutherford's Clinical Lectures in Edinburgh, 1749–53." *Journal of the History of Medicine and Allied Sciences* 72, no. 3 (2017): 302–27.

Crellin, J. K. "Early Settlements in Newfoundland and the Scourge of Scurvy." *Canadian Bulletin of the History of Medicine* 17 (2000): 127–36.

Cross, Anthony. *By the Banks of the Neva: Chapters from the Lives and Careers of the British in Eighteenth-Century Russia*. New York: Cambridge University Press, 1997.

Cross, Anthony. "Chaplains to the British Factory in St. Petersburg, 1723–1813." *European History Quarterly* 2, no. 2 (1972): 125–42.

Cross, Anthony. "The Reverend William Tooke's Contribution to English Knowledge of Russia at the End of the Eighteenth Century." *Canadian Slavic Studies* 3, no. 1 (1969): 106–15.

Culver, Lawrence. "The Desert and the Garden: Climate as Attractor and Obstacle in the Settlement History of the Western United States." *Global Environment* 5, no. 9 (2012): 130–59.

Cunningham, Andrew. "Medicine to Calm the Mind: Boerhaave's Medical System, and Why It Was Adopted in Edinburgh." In *The Medical Enlightenment of the Eighteenth Century*, edited by Andrew Cunningham and Roger French, 40–66. New York: Cambridge University Press, 1990.

Curran, Andrew S. *The Anatomy of Blackness: Science and Slavery in an Age of Enlightenment*. Baltimore, MD: Johns Hopkins University Press, 2011.

Dainotto, Roberto M. *Europe (In Theory)*. Durham, NC: Duke University Press, 2007.

Daston, Lorraine. "The Ideal and Reality of the Republic of Letters in the Enlightenment." *Science in Context* 4, no. 2 (1991): 367–86.

Daston, Lorraine, and Elizabeth Lunbeck, eds. *Histories of Scientific Observation*. Chicago: University of Chicago Press, 2011.

Debus, Allen G. "Chemists, Physicians, and Changing Perspectives on the Scientific Revolution." *Isis* 89, no. 1 (1998): 66–81.

DeLacy, Margaret. "The Conceptualization of Influenza in Eighteenth-Century Britain: Specificity and Contagion." *Bulletin of the History of Medicine* 67, no. 1 (1993): 74–118.

DeLacy, Margaret. *The Germ of an Idea: Contagionism, Religion, and Society in Britain, 1660–1730*. New York: Palgrave Macmillan, 2016.

DeLacy, Margaret. "Nosology, Mortality, and Disease Theory in the Eighteenth Century." *Journal of the History of Medicine and Allied Sciences* 54, no. 2 (1999): 261–84.

Dimsdale, Robert. "Mixed Blessing: The Impact of Suttonian Smallpox Inoculation in the Later Eighteenth Century." *SGECR Occasional Series* 1. Accessed July 12, 2022. https://www.sgecr.co.uk/dimsdale/article.html.

Dmytryshyn, Basil. "Iurii Krizhanich: The First Sibirologist." *Russian History* 18, no. 2 (1991): 143–61.

Donkin, R. A. *Manna: An Historical Geography*. The Hague: Kluwer Academic, 1980.

Dorwart, Reinhold A. "The Royal College of Medicine and Public Health in Brandenburg-Prussia, 1685–1740." *Medical History* 2, no. 1 (1958): 13–23.

Douglas, Bronwen. "Slippery Word, Ambiguous Practice: 'Race' and Late-18th-Century Voyagers in Oceania." *Journal of Pacific History* 41, no. 1 (2006): 1–29.

Driessen van het Reve, Jozien J. "Hoe Nicolaas Bidloo (1673/4–1735) de medische cultuur van Amsterdam naar Moskou bracht." *Mededelingen van de Stichting Jacob Campo Weyerman* 34 (2011): 5–22.

Driessen van het Reve, Jozien. "Peter the Great and His Dutch Teachers." In *Peter the Great: An Inspired Tsar*, edited by Mikhail Piotrovsky and Cathelijne Broers, 150–53. Amsterdam: Heritage Amsterdam, 2013.

Dunlap, Barbara J. "The Problem of Syphilitic Children in Eighteenth-Century France and England." In *The Secret Malady: Venereal Disease in Eighteenth-Century Britain and France*, edited by Linda E. Merians, 114–27. Lexington: University Press of Kentucky, 1996.

Earle, Rebecca. *The Body of the Conquistador: Food, Race and the Colonial Experience in Spanish America, 1492–1700*. New York: Cambridge University Press, 2012.

Easterby-Smith, Sarah. "Reputation in a Box: Objects, Communication and Trust in Late 18th-Century Botanical Networks." *History of Science* 53, no. 2 (2015): 180–208.

Ehninger, Douglas. "On Systems of Rhetoric." *Philosophy and Rhetoric* 25 (1992): 15–28.

Emch-Dériaz, Antoinette. "The Non-Naturals Made Easy." In *The Popularization of Medicine, 1650–1850*, edited by Roy Porter, 134–59. London: Routledge, 1992.

Epatko, Yury G. "James Mounsey: A Scot in the Service of Russia." *Scottish Slavonic Review* 4 (1985): 7–9.

Erikson, Gunnar. "Linnaeus the Botanist." In *Linnaeus: The Man and His Work*. edited by Tore Frängmyr, 63–94. Berkeley: University of California Press, 1983.

Evangulova, O. S. "Rukopisi N. Bidloo v sobranii biblioteki Rossiiskoi Akademii Nauk (K istorii panegiricheskogo napraveleniia v russkoi kul'ture petrovskogo vremeni)." *Vestnik Moskovskogo universiteta*, Seriia 8: *Istoriia* 3 (2000): 68–86.

Fagan, Brian M. *The Little Ice Age: How Climate Made History, 1300–1850*. New York: Basic, 2001.

Foust, Clifford M. *Muscovite and Mandarin: Russia's Trade with China and Its Setting, 1727–1805*. Chapel Hill: University of North Carolina Press, 1969.

Frängsmyr, Tore, ed. *Linnaeus: The Man and His Work*. Berkeley: University of California Press, 1983.

Frost, Orcutt. "Georg Steller and Stepan Krasheninnikov: Pioneer Scholars on the North Pacific Rim." *Pacific Northwest Quarterly* 95, no. 2 (2004): 59–69.

Frost, Orcutt. "Vitus Bering and Georg Steller: Their Tragic Conflict During the American Expedition." *Pacific Northwest Quarterly* 86, no. 1 (1994/1995): 3–16.

Gallagher, Noelle. *Itch, Clap, Pox: Venereal Disease in the Eighteenth-Century Imagination*. New Haven, CT: Yale University Press, 2018.

Gänger, Stephanie. "World Trade in Medicinal Plants from Spanish America, 1717-1815." *Medical History* 59:1 (2015): 44–82.

Gascoigne, John. "The Royal Society, Natural History and the Peoples of the 'New World(s),' 1660–1800." *British Journal for the History of Science* 42, no. 4 (2009): 539–62.

Geertz, Clifford. *The Interpretation of Cultures*. New York: Basic, 1973.

Gelfand, Toby. *Professionalizing Modern Medicine: Paris Surgeons and Medical Science and Institutions in the 18th Century*. Westport, CT: Greenwood, 1980.

Geyer-Kordesch, Johanna. "German Medical Education in the Eighteenth Century: The Prussian Context and Its Influence." In *William Hunter and the Eighteenth-Century Medical World*, edited by W. F. Bynum and Roy Porter, 177–205. New York: Cambridge University Press, 1985.

Gibson, James R. *Feeding the Russian Fur Trade: Provisionment of the Okhotsk Seaboard and the Kamchatka Peninsula, 1639–1856*. Madison: University of Wisconsin Press, 1969.

Gómez, Pablo F. *The Experimental Caribbean: Creating Knowledge and Healing in the Early Modern Atlantic*. Chapel Hill: University of North Carolina Press, 2017.

Gordin, Michael D. "The Importation of Being Earnest: The Early St. Petersburg Academy of Sciences." *Isis* 91, no. 1 (2000): 1–31.

Goslings, W. R. O. "Leiden and Edinburgh: The Seed, the Soil and the Climate." In *The Early Years of the Edinburgh Medical School*, edited by R. G. W. Anderson and A. D. C. Simpson, 1–16. Edinburgh: Royal Scottish Museum, 1976.

Gouzévitch, Dmitri. "The Delisle Brothers in Russia: Victims of Historiography and Scurvy." In *In Foreign Lands: The Migrations of Scientists for Political or Economic Reason*, edited by Maria Teresa Borgato and Christine Phili, 55–84. Basel: Birkhauser, 2022.

Griffin, Clare. "In Search of an Audience: Popular Pharmacies and the Limits of Literate Medicine in Late Seventeenth- and Early Eighteenth-Century Russia." *Bulletin of the History of Medicine* 89, no. 4 (2015): 705–32.

Griffin, Clare. *Mixing Medicines: The Global Drug Trade and Early Modern Russia*. Montreal: McGill-Queen's University Press, 2022.

Griffin, Clare. "Russia and the Medical Drug Trade in the Seventeenth Century." *Social History of Medicine* 31, no. 1 (2018): 2–23.

Grinëv, Andrei V. "Anglo-Russian Rivalry in the American Arctic, Eighteenth to Mid-Nineteenth Centuries." *Northern Review* 49 (2020): 167–90.

Grinëv, Andrei V. "Reflections on the Fate of Alexei Chirikov's Missing Men." Translated by Richard L. Bland. *Arctic Anthropology* 42, no. 2 (2005): 1–8.

Grinëv, Andrei V. "Russian Maritime Catastrophes During the Colonization of Alaska, 1741–1867." Translated by Richard L. Bland. *Pacific Northwest Quarterly* 102, no. 4 (2011): 178–94.

Grinëv, Andrei V. *The Tlingit Indians in Russian America, 1741–1867*. Translated by Richard L. Bland and Katerina G. Solovjova. Lincoln: University of Nebraska Press, 2005.

Grmek, Mirko. "The History of Medical Education in Russia." In *The History of Medical Education*, edited by C. D. O'Malley, 303–28. Berkeley: University of California Press, 1970.

Grombakh, S. M. *Russkaia meditsinskaia literatura XVIII veka*. Moscow: Izdatel'stvo Akademii meditsinskikh nauk SSSR, 1953.

Gunther, Albert E. "Edward Whitaker Gray (1748–1806): Keeper of Natural Curiosities at the British Museum." *Bulletin of the British Museum (Natural History)* 5, no. 2 (1976): 191–210.

Guzevich, D. and I. Guzevich. *Velikoe posol'stvo*. St. Petersburg: Feniks, 2003.

Haigh, Basil. "Design for a Medical Service: Peter the Great's Admiralty Regulations (1722)." *Medical History* 19 (1975): 129–46.

Hans, Nicholas. "Russian Students at Leyden in the 18th Century." *Slavonic and East European Review* 35 (1957): 551–62.

Harrison, Mark. *Climates and Constitutions: Health, Race, Environment and British Imperialism in India, 1600–1850*. New York: Oxford University Press, 1999.

Harrison, Mark. *Medicine in an Age of Commerce and Empire: Britain and Its Tropical Colonies, 1660–1830*. New York: Oxford University Press, 2010.

Headrick, Daniel R. *When Information Came of Age: Technologies of Knowledge in the Age of Reason and Revolution, 1700–1850*. New York: Oxford University Press, 2000.

Herbert, Amanda E. "Gender and the Spa: Space, Sociability and Self at the British Health Spas, 1640–1714." *Journal of Social History* 43, no. 2 (2009): 361–83.

Herzberg. Julia. "Climate Ideas and the Cold in Russia." In *The Russian Cold: Histories of Ice, Frost, and Snow*, edited by Julia Herzberg, Andreas Renner, and Ingrid Schierle, 19–43. New York: Berghahn, 2021.

Herzberg, Julia. "The Nature of Cold: Russia's Climate and the Academy of Sciences in the Eighteenth Century." In *The Russian Cold: Histories of Ice, Frost, and Snow*, edited by Julia Herzberg, Andreas Renner, and Ingrid Schierle, 47–73. New York: Berghahn, 2021.

Herzberg, Julia, Andreas Renner, and Ingrid Schierle, eds. *The Russian Cold: Histories of Ice, Frost, and Snow*. New York: Berghahn, 2021.

Heuvel, Charles van den, Scott B. Weingart, Nils Spelt, and Henk Nellen. "Circles of Confidence in Correspondence: Modeling Confidentiality and Secrecy in Knowledge Exchange Networks of Letters and Drawings in the Early Modern Period." *Nuncius* 31 (2016): 78–106.

Hodacs, Hanna. "Linnaeans Outdoors: The Transformative Role of Studying Nature 'on the Move' and Outside." *British Journal for the History of Science* 44, no. 2 (2011): 183–209.

Hoffmann, Peter. "Strahlenberg, Philipp Johann von," In *Neue Deutsche Biographie*, Band 25. Berlin: Duncker & Humblot, 2013. 464–65.

Hogarth, Rana A. *Medicalizing Blackness: Making Racial Difference in the Atlantic World, 1780–1840*. Chapel Hill: University of North Carolina Press, 2017.

Hudson, Nicholas. "From 'Nation' to 'Race': The Origin of Racial Classification in Eighteenth-Century Thought." *Eighteenth-Century Studies* 29, no. 3 (1996): 247–64.

Hughes, R. E. "James Lind and the Cure of Scurvy: An Experimental Approach." *Medical History* 19 (1975): 342–51.

Hunter, Michael, and Edward B. Davis. "The Making of Robert Boyle's 'Free Enquiry Into the Vulgary Receiv'd Notion of Nature' (1686)." *Early Science and Medicine* 1, no. 2 (1996): 204–71.

Ippolitova, A. B. *Russkie pukopisnye travniki XVII-XVIII vekov: Issledovanie fol'klora i etnobotaniki*. Moscow: Indrik, 2008.

Jennings, Henry. "The Boundaries of Eurasia: Dividing Lands, Minds, and Bodies in Eighteenth-Century Siberia." *Sibirica* 21, no. 1 (2022): 53–78.

Jones, Peter M. *Agricultural Enlightenment: Knowledge, Technology, and Nature, 1750–1840*. New York: Oxford University Press, 2016.

Jones, Ryan Tucker. *Empire of Extinction: Russians and the North Pacific's Strange Beasts of the Sea, 1741–1867*. New York: Oxford University Press, 2014.

Jones, Ryan Tucker. "Peter Simon Pallas, Siberia, and the European Republic of Letters." *Istoriko-biologicheskie issledovaniia* 3, no. 3 (2011): 55-67.

Jütte, Robert. "The Social Construction of Illness in the Early Modern Period." In *The Social Construction of Illness: Illness and Medical Knowledge in Past and Present*, edited by Jens Lachmund and Gunnar Stollberg, 23-38. Stuttgart: Franz Steiner Verlag, 1992.

Kananoja, Kalle. *Healing Knowledge in Atlantic Africa: Medical Encounters, 1500–1850*. New York: Cambridge University Press, 2021.

Kelton, Paul. *Cherokee Medicine, Colonial Germs: An Indigenous Nation's Fight Against Smallpox, 1518–1824*. Norman: University of Oklahoma Press, 2015.

Kidd, Colin. *The Forging of Races: Race and Scripture in the Protestant Atlantic World, 1600–2000*. New York: Cambridge University Press, 2006.

Kivelson, Valerie. "'The Devil Stole His Mind': The Tsar and the 1648 Moscow Uprising." *American Historical Review* 98, no. 3 (1993): 733-56.

Kirillov, V. V. "Moskva iauzskaia (K rekonstruktsii pervykh gospital'nykh zdanii petrovskogo vremenii i usad'by N. Bidloo)." *Vestnik Moskovskogo universiteta*, Seriia 8: *Istoriia* 1 (2001): 93-103.

Klein, Ursula. "The Laboratory Challenge: Some Revisions of the Standard View of Early Modern Experimentation." *Isis* 99, no. 4 (2008): 769-82.

Knoppers, Jake V. Th. "The Visits of Peter the Great to the United Provinces in 1697-1698 and 1716-1717 as Seen in Light of the Dutch Sources." Master's thesis, McGill University, 1969.

Koerner, Lisbet. *Linnaeus: Nature and Nation*. Cambridge, MA: Harvard University Press, 1999.

Konczacki, Zbigniew A. "Economic and Social Thought in Poland During the Period Between Partitions (1772-1795)." *Polish Review* 39, no. 2 (1994): 169-83.

Koroloff, Rachel. "'In Imperio Rutheno': Johann Amman's *Stirpium rariorum* (1739) and the Foundation of Russia's Botanical Empire." In *The Botany of Empire in the Long Eighteenth Century*, edited by Yota Batsaki, Sarah Burke Cahalan, and Anatole Tchikine, 235-56. Washington, DC: Dumbarton Oaks Research Library, 2016.

Kowal, Areta O. "Danilo Samoilowitz: An Eighteenth-Century Ukrainian Epidemiologist and His Role in the Moscow Plague (1770–72)." *Journal of the History of Medicine and Applied Sciences* 27 (1972): 434-46.

Kowner, Rowtem. *From White to Yellow: The Japanese in European Racial Thought, 1300–1735*. Montreal: McGill-Queen's University Press, 2014.

Küçük, Harun. *Science Without Leisure: Practical Naturalism in Istanbul, 1660–1732*. Pittsburgh: University of Pittsburgh Press, 2020.

Kuentzel-Witt, Kristina. "Eisfrei über den Nordpol? Die Suche nach der Nordostpassage im 18. Jh." *Osteuropa* 70, no. 5 (2020): 23-37.

Kuentzel-Witt, Kristina. "Peter the Great's Intermezzo with G. W. Liebniz and G. Delisle: The Development of Geographical Knowledge in Russia." *Quaestio Rossica* 6, no. 1 (2018): 63-78.

Kupperman, Karen Ordahl. "Fear of Hot Climates in the Anglo-American Colonial Experience." *William and Mary Quarterly*, 3rd ser., vol. 41, no. 2 (1984): 213–40.

Kupperman, Karen Ordahl. "The Puzzle of the American Climate in the Early Colonial Period." *American Historical Review* 87, no. 5 (1982): 1262–89.

Kuxhausen, Anna. *From the Womb to the Body Politic: Raising the Nation in Enlightenment Russia*. Madison: University of Wisconsin Press, 2013.

Larson, James L. *Reason and Experience: The Representation of Natural Order in the World of Carl von Linné*. Berkeley: University of California Press, 1971.

Lamb, Jonathan. *Preserving the Self in the South Seas, 1680–1840*. Chicago: University of Chicago Press, 2001.

Lamb, Jonathan. "The Rime of the Ancient Mariner: A Ballad of Scurvy." In *Pathologies of Travel*, edited by Richard Wrigley and George Revill, 157–77. Amsterdam: Rodopoi, 2000.

Lees, Lynn Holland. *Planting Empire, Cultivating Subjects: British Malaya, 1786–1941*. New York: Cambridge University Press, 2017.

Leete, Art. "Silence in the Woods: Finno-Ugric Peoples of the Russian North and Western Siberia in the Ethnographic Literature from the Eighteenth to the Twentieth Century." *Sibirica* 18, no. 2 (2019): 1–26.

Levitt, Marcus C. "An Antidote to Nervous Juice: Catherine the Great's Debate with Chappe d'Auteroche Over Russian Culture." *Eighteenth-Century Studies* 32, no. 1 (1998): 49–63.

Lindeboom, G. A. *Herman Boerhaave: The Man and His Work*. London: Methuen, 1968.

Lindroth, Sten. "The Two Faces of Linnaeus." In *Linnaeus: The Man and His Work*, edited by Tore Frängsmyr, 1–62. Berkeley: University of California Press, 1983.

Liubimenko, Inna. "Vrachebnoe i lekarstvennoe delo v Moskovskom gosudartsv." *Russkii istoricheskie zhurnal* 1, no. 3–4 (1917): 1–36.

Loewensen, Leo. "People Peter Met in England." *Slavonic and East European Review* 37 (1959): 459–68.

Loewenson, Leo. "The Works of Robert Boyle and 'The Present State of Russia' by Samuel Collins (1671)." *Slavonic and East European Review* 33 (1955): 470–85.

Lomax, Elizabeth. "Difficulties in Diagnosing Infantile Scurvy before 1878." *Medical History*, 30 (1986): 70–80.

Louis-Courvoisier, Micheline, and Alexandre Mauron. " 'He found me very well; for me, I was still feeling sick': The Strange Worlds of Physicians and Patients in the 18th and 21st Centuries." *Journal of Medical Ethics: Medical Humanities* 28 (2002): 9–13.

Lux, David S., and Harold J. Cook. "Closed Circles or Open Networks? Communicating at a Distance During the Scientific Revolution." *History of Science* 36 (1998): 179–211.

Manen, Niels van. "Preventative Medicine in the Dutch Slave Trade, 1747–1797." *International Journal of Maritime History* 18, no. 2 (2006): 129–85.

Mattson, Greggor. "Nation-State Science: Lappology and Sweden's Ethnoracial Purity." *Comparative Studies in Society and History* 56, no. 2 (2014): 320–50.

Mazierski, David M. "The Cabinet of Frederick Ruysch and the Kunstkamera of Peter the Great: Past and Present." *Journal of Biocommunication* 38 (2012): E31–E40.

McClellan, James E. *Colonialism and Science: Saint Domingue in the Old Regime*. Chicago: University of Chicago Press, 1992.

Merrens, H. Roy, and George D. Terry. "Dying in Paradise: Malaria, Mortality, and the Perpetual Environment in Colonial South Carolina." *Journal of Southern History* 50, no. 4 (1984): 533–50.

Miller, Genevieve. *The Adoption of Inoculation for Smallpox in England and France*. Philadelphia: University of Pennsylvania Press, 1957.

Miller, Genevieve. "'Airs, Waters, and Places' in History." *Journal of the History of Medicine and the Allied Sciences* 17 (1962): 129–38.

Miller, Gwen A. *Kodiak Kreol: Communities of Empire in Early Russian America*. Ithaca, NY: Cornell University Press, 2010.

Mirskii, M. B. "Moscow Hospital School." *Medicina nei Secoli Arte e Scienza* 3 (1991): 233–41.

Monahan, Erika. *The Merchants of Siberia: Trade in Early Modern Russia*. Ithaca, NY: Cornell University Press, 2016.

Morgan, Jennifer L. *Laboring Women: Reproduction and Gender in New World Slavery*. Philadelphia: University of Pennsylvania Press, 2004.

Murdoch, Steve. *Network North: Scottish Kin, Commercial and Covert Associations in Northern Europe, 1603–1746*. Leiden: Brill, 2006.

Napol'skikh, V. V. *Udmurtskie materialy D. G. Messershmidta: Dnevnikovye zapisi, dekabr' 1726*. Izhevsk: Udmurtiia, 2001.

Natochin, Iu. V. "Stanovlenie fiziologii v Rossii: XVIII vek." *Istoriko-biologicheskie issledovaniia* 8, no. 2 (2016): 9–24.

Newton, Gill. "Diagnosing Rickets in Early Modern England: Statistical Evidence and Social Response." *Social History of Medicine* 35, no. 2 (2022): 566–88.

Olwig, Kenneth Robert. *Landscape, Nature, and the Body Politic: From Britain's Renaissance to America's New World*. Madison: University of Wisconsin Press, 2002.

O'Neill, Lindsay. *The Opened Letter: Networking in the Early Modern British World*. Philadelphia: University of Pennsylvania Press, 2015.

Okenfuss, Max J. "Catherine, Montesquieu, and Empire." *Jahrbücher für Geschichte Osteuropas* 56, no. 3 (2008): 322–29.

Papmehl, K. A. "Matthew Guthrie: The Forgotten Student of 18th Century Russia." *Canadian Slavonic Papers* 11, no. 2 (1969): 167–81.

Parker, Geoffrey. *Global Crisis: War, Climate Change, and Catastrophe in the Seventeenth Century*. New Haven, CT: Yale University Press, 2013.

Paul, Robert. "Scotsmen in Russian Service." *The Scotsman*, August 31, 1895.

Pender, Stephen, and Nancy S. Struever, eds. *Rhetoric and Medicine in Early Modern Europe*. Farnham, Surrey: Ashgate, 2012.

Petrov, B. D. "Tsinga i bor'ba s nei v Rossii." *Voprosy pitaniia* 17, no. 4 (1958): 78–83.

Piper, Liza. *When Disease Came to This Country: Epidemics and Colonialism in Northern North America*. New York: Cambridge University Press, 2023.

Poe, Marshall T. *"A People Born to Slavery": Russia in Early Modern European Ethnography, 1476–1748*. Ithaca, NY: Cornell University Press, 2000.

Pokrovskii, N. N. *Tomsk 1648–1649 gg.: Voevodskaia vlast' i zemskie mir*. Novosibirsk: Nauka, 1989.

Pollock, Ethan. *Without the Banya We Would Perish: A History of the Russian Bathhouse*. New York: Oxford University Press, 2019.

Porter, Roy "The Early Royal Society and the Spread of Medical Knowledge." In *The Medical Revolution of the Seventeenth Century*, edited by Roger French and Andrew Wear, 272–93. New York: Cambridge University Press, 1989.

Porter, Roy. "Was There a Medical Enlightenment in Eighteenth-Century England?" *British Journal of Eighteenth-Century Studies* 5, no. 1 (1982): 49–63.

Pratt, Mary Louise. *Imperial Eyes: Travel Writing and Transculturation*. 2nd ed. New York: Routledge, 2008.

Purdue, Peter C. "Boundaries, Maps, and Movement: Chinese, Russian, and Mongolian Empires in Early Modern Central Eurasia." *International History Review* 20, no. 2 (1998): 263–86.

Radvoskii, M. I. "U istokov anglo-russkikh nauchnykh sviazei." *Istoricheskii arkhiv* 3 (1956): 139–55.

Raj, Kapil. *Relocating Modern Science: Circulation and the Construction of Knowledge in South Asia and Europe, 1650–1800*. London: Palgrave Macmillan, 2007.

Reis, Elizabeth. "Impossible Hermaphrodites: Intersex in America, 1620–1960." *Journal of American History* 92, no. 2 (2005): 411–41.

Riley, James C. "The Medicine of the Environment in Eighteenth-Century Germany." *Clio Medica* 18 (1983): 167–78.

Risse, Guenter B. "Clinical Instruction in Hospitals: The Boerhaavian Tradition in Leyden, Edinburgh, Vienna and Pavia." *Clio Medica* 21 (1987–1988): 1–19.

Robarts, Andrew. *Migration and Disease in the Black Sea Region: Ottoman-Russian Relations in the Late Eighteenth and Early Nineteenth Centuries*. London: Bloomsbury Academic, 2017.

Romaniello, Matthew P. "Commodities with Context: Moving Materials and Medical Knowledge into Medieval Russia." *Canadian-American Slavic Studies* 57, no. 3–4 (2023): 468–83.

Romaniello, Matthew P. "Could Siberian 'Natural Curiosities' Be Replaced? Biosprospecting in the Eighteenth Century." *Early Science and Medicine* 27, no. 3 (2022): 257–77.

Romaniello, Matthew P. *Enterprising Empires: Russia and Britain in Eighteenth-Century Eurasia*. New York: Cambridge University Press, 2019.

Romaniello, Matthew P. "Humoral Bodies in Cold Climates." In *Russian History through the Senses: From 1700 to the Present*, edited by Matthew P. Romaniello and Tricia Starks, 23–43. London: Bloomsbury, 2016.

Rosner, Lisa. *Medical Education in the Age of Improvement: Edinburgh Students and Apprentices, 1760–1826*. Edinburgh: Edinburgh University Press, 1991.

Ross, Corey. *Ecology and Power in the Age of Empire: Europe and the Transformation of the Tropical World*. New York: Oxford University Press, 2017.

Rowell, Margery. "Linnaeus and Botanists in Eighteenth-Century Russia." *Taxon* 29, no. 1 (1980): 15–26.

Rubiés, Joan-Pau. "Oriental Despotism and European Orientalism: Botero to Montesquieu." *Journal of Early Modern History* 9, no. 1–2 (2005): 109–80.

Rusnock, Andrea. "Correspondence Networks and the Royal Society, 1700–1750." *British Journal for the History of Science* 32, no. 2 (1999): 155–69.

Rutman, Darrett B., and Anita H. Rutman. "Of Agues and Fevers: Malaria in the Early Chesapeake." *William and Mary Quarterly*, 3rd ser., 33, no. 1 (1976): 31–60.

Savel'eva, E. A., ed. *Katalog knig iz sobraniia aptekarskogo prikaza*. St. Petersburg: Al'faret, 2006.

Schiebinger, Londa. *Nature's Body: Gender in the Making of Modern Science*. New Brunswick, NJ: Rutgers University Press, 2004.

Schiebinger, Londa. *Plants and Empire: Colonial Bioprospecting in the Atlantic World*. Cambridge, MA: Harvard University Press, 2004.

Schiebinger, Londa. *Secret Cures of Slaves: People, Plants, and Medicine in the Eighteenth-Century Atlantic World*. Stanford, CA: Stanford University Press, 2017.

Schiebinger, Londa. "Why Mammals Are Called Mammals: Gender Politics in Eighteenth-Century Natural History." *American Historical Review* 98, no. 2 (1993): 382–411.

Seth, Suman. *Difference and Disease: Medicine, Race, and the Eighteenth-Century British Empire*. New York: Cambridge University Press, 2018.

Seth, Vanita. *Europe's Indians: Producing Racial Difference, 1500–1900*. Durham, NC: Duke University Press, 2010.

Shishilov, I. A. "K istorii izucheniia materialov S. P. Krasheninnikov: Problemy, diskussii, novye informatsiia i interpretatsii." *Gumanitarnye nauki v Sibiri* 25, no. 3 (2018), 64–8.

Shoemaker, Nancy. "How Indians Got to Be Red." *American Historical Review* 102, no. 3 (1997): 625–44.

Siena, Kevin P. *Venereal Disease, Hospitals, and the Urban Poor: London's "Foul Wards," 1600–1800*. Rochester, NY: University of Rochester Press, 2004.

Simonov, R. A. "Iatronauchnyi etap Russkoi estestvenno-nauchnoi knizhnost (nachalo XVIII vv.)." *Voprosy istorii estestvoznaiia i tekhniki* 1 (2007): 58–89.

Sköld, Peter. "Escape from Catastrophe: The Saami's Experience with Smallpox in Eighteenth- and Nineteenth-Century Sweden." *Social Science History* 21, no. 1 (1997): 1–25.

Skott, Christina. "Human Taxonomies: Carl Linnaeus, Swedish Travel in Asia and the Classification of Man." *Itinerario* 43, no. 2 (2019): 218–42.

Slezkine, Yuri. *Arctic Mirrors: Russian and the Small Peoples of the North*. Ithaca, NY: Cornell University Press, 1994,

Slezkine, Yuri. "The Sovereign's Foreigners: Classifying the Native Peoples in Seventeenth-Century Siberia." *Russian History* 19 (1992): 475–85.

Sloan, Phillip R. "Buffon, German Biology, and the Historical Interpretation of Biological Species." *British Journal for the History of Science* 12, no. 2 (1979): 109–53.

Smith, Alison K. "'The Freedom to Choose a Way of Life': Fugitives, Borders, and Imperial Amnesties in Russia." *Journal of Modern History* 83 (2011): 243–71.

Smith, Alison K. "Movement and the Transformation of Siberia in the Eighteenth Century." *Sibirica* 16, no. 2 (2017): 44–67.

Ssu-ming, Meng. "The E-lo-ssu kuan (Russian Hostel) in Peking." *Harvard Journal of Asiatic Studies* 23 (1960–61): 19–46.

Stearn, William T. "The Influence of Leyden on Botany in the Seventeenth and Eighteenth Centuries." *British Journal for the History of Science* 1, no. 2 (1962): 137–58.

Stein, Claudia. *Negotiating the French Pox in Early Modern Germany*. Farnham, Surrey: Ashgate, 2009.

Stevens, Roger. "John Bell of Antermony, and His Travels in Iran." *Iran* 16 (1978): 177–82.

Stolberg, Eva-Maria. "Interracial Outposts in Siberia: Nerchinsk, Kiakhta, and the Russo-Chinese Trade in the Seventeenth/Eighteenth Centuries." *Journal of Early Modern History* 4, no. 3–4 (2000): 322–36.

Sundberg, Adam. *Natural Disaster at the Closing of the Dutch Golden Age: Floods, Worms, and Cattle Plagues*. Cambridge: Cambridge University Press, 2022.

Taki, Victor. "Orientalism on the Margins: The Ottoman Empire under Russian Eyes." *Kritika* 12, no. 2 (2011): 321–51.

Tansey, E. M. "The Life and Works of Sir Alexander Crichton, F.R.S. (1763–1856): A Scotsman Physician to the Imperial Russian Court." *Notes and Records of the Royal Society of London* 38, no. 2 (1984): 241–59.

Thomas, Christine J. "Sir Hans Sloane and the Russian Academy of Sciences." *British Library Journal* 14, no. 1 (1988): 21–37.

Titova, Z. D. "Puteshestvie po ukazu Petra I: Iz dnevnika D. G. Messershmidta—Issledovatelia narodov Sibiri, 1721–1725 gg." *Istoricheskii arkhiv* 2 (2003): 21–40.

Toropitsyn, I. V. "Vliiane karantinnykh meropriiatii na sostoianie russko-vostochnoi torgovli i torgovogosudokhodstva v Kaspiiskom basseine vo vtoroi cheverti XVIII veka." *Vestnik Samaraskogo gosudarstvennogo universiteta* 69, no. 3 (2009): 95–100.

Unkovskaya, Maria V. *Brief Lives: A Handbook of Medical Practitioners in Muscovy, 1620–1701*. London: Wellcome Library, 1999.

Varlik, Nükhet. *Plague and Empire in the Early Modern Mediterranean World: The Ottoman Experience, 1347–1600*. New York: Cambridge University Press, 2015.

Vermeulen, Han F. *Before Boas: The Genesis of Ethnography and Ethnology in the German Enlightenment*. Lincoln: University of Nebraska Press, 2015.

Vinkovetsky, Ilya. "Circumnavigation, Empire, Modernity, Race: The Impact of Round-the-World Voyages on Russia's Imperial Consciousness." *Ab Imperio* 1, no. 2 (2001): 191–209.

Vinkovetsky, Ilya. *Russian America: An Overseas Colony of a Continental Empire, 1804–1867*. New York: Oxford University Press, 2011.

Warde, Paul. *The Invention of Sustainability: Nature and Destiny, c. 1500–1870*. New York: Cambridge University Press, 2018.

Weightman, Gavin. *The Great Inoculator: The Untold Story of Daniel Sutton and His Medical Revolution*. New Haven, CT: Yale University Press, 2020.

Weisser, Olivia. "Treating the Secret Disease: Sex, Sin, and Authority in Eighteenth-Century Venereal Cases." *Bulletin of the History of Medicine* 91, no. 4 (2017): 685–712.

Werrett, Simon. "The Schumacher Affair: Reconfiguring Academic Expertise Across Dynasties in Eighteenth-Century Russia." *Osiris* 25, no.1 (2010): 104–26.

Wilms, Sabine. "'Ten Times More Difficult to Treat': Female Bodies in Medical Texts from Early Imperial China." In *Medicine for Women in Imperial China*, edited by Angela Ki Che Leung, 74–107. Leiden: Brill, 2006.

Winston, Michael. "Medicine, Marriage, and Human Degeneration in the French Enlightenment." *Eighteenth-Century Studies* 38, no. 2 (2005): 263–81.

Wisecup, Kelly. *Medical Encounters: Knowledge and Identity in Early American Literature*. Amherst: University of Massachusetts Press, 2013.

Wolfe, Patrick. *Settler Colonialism and the Transformation of Anthropology: The Politics and Poetics of an Ethnographic Event*. London: Cassell, 1999.

Wolff, Larry. *Inventing Eastern Europe: The Map of Civilization on the Mind of Enlightenment*. Stanford, CA: Stanford University Press, 1994.

Wortman, Richard. "Texts of Exploration and Russia's European Identity." In *Visual Texts, Ceremonial Texts, and Texts of Exploration: Collected Articles on the Representation of the Russian Monarchy*, 253–73. Brighton, MA: Academic Studies, 2014.

Yang, Bin. "The Zhang on Chinese Southern Frontiers: Disease Constructions, Environmental Changes, and Imperial Colonization." *Bulletin of the History of Medicine* 84, no. 2 (2010): 163–92.

Zeheter, Michael. *Epidemics, Empire, and Environments: Cholera in Madras and Quebec City, 1818–1910*. Pittsburgh: University of Pittsburgh Press, 2015.

Zilberstein, Anya. *A Temperate Empire: Making Climate Change in Early America*. New York: Oxford University Press, 2016.

Znamenski, Andrei A. "History with an Attitude: Alaska in Modern Russian Patriotic Rhetoric." *Jahrbücher für Geschichte Osteuropas* 57 (2009): 346–73.

Index

www.ingramcontent.com/pod-product-compliance
Lightning Source LLC
Chambersburg PA
CBHW020142061025
33560CB00038B/6
9781501783920